MEDICAL IMAGING

MEDICAL IMAGING

Harry LeVine, III

Health and Medical Issues Today

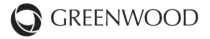
GREENWOOD

AN IMPRINT OF ABC-CLIO, LLC
Santa Barbara, California • Denver, Colorado • Oxford, England

Copyright 2010 by Harry LeVine, III

Library of Congress Cataloging-in-Publication Data
Medical imaging / Harry LeVine, III.
    p. cm.—(Health and medical issues today)
  Includes bibliographical references and index.
  ISBN 978-0-313-35969-9 (hard copy : alk. paper)—ISBN 978-0-313-
35970-5 (ebook) 1. Diagnostic imaging. I. LeVine, Harry, 1949–
  RC78.7.D53M4283   2010
  616.07′54—dc22   2009050076

ISBN: 978-0-313-35969-9
EISBN: 978-0-313-35970-5

14 13 12 11 10   1 2 3 4 5

This book is also available on the World Wide Web as an eBook.
Visit www.abc-clio.com for details.

Greenwood
An Imprint of ABC-CLIO, LLC

ABC-CLIO, LLC
130 Cremona Drive, P.O. Box 1911
Santa Barbara, California 93116-1911

This book is printed on acid-free paper ∞

Manufactured in the United States of America

CONTENTS

SERIES FOREWORD

Every day, the public is bombarded with information on developments in medicine and health care. Whether it is on the latest techniques in treatments or research, or on concerns over public health threats, this information directly affects the lives of people more than almost any other issue. Although there are many sources for understanding these topics— from Web sites and blogs to newspapers and magazines—students and ordinary citizens often need one resource that makes sense of the complex health and medical issues affecting their daily lives.

The *Health and Medical Issues Today* series provides just such a one-stop resource for obtaining a solid overview of the most controversial areas of health care in the twenty-first century. Each volume addresses one topic and provides a balanced summary of what is known. These volumes provide an excellent first step for students and lay people interested in understanding how health care works in our society today.

Each volume is broken into several sections to provide readers and researchers with easy access to the information they need:

- Section I provides overview chapters on background information—including chapters on such areas as the historical, scientific, medical, social, and legal issues involved—that a citizen needs to intelligently understand the topic.
- Section II provides capsule examinations of the most heated contemporary issues and debates, and analyzes in a balanced manner the viewpoints held by various advocates in the debates.

- Section III provides a selection of reference material, such as annotated primary source documents, a timeline of important events, and a directory of organizations that serve as the best next step in learning about the topic at hand.

The *Health and Medical Issues Today* series strives to provide readers with all the information needed to begin making sense of some of the most important debates going on in the world today. The series includes volumes on such topics as stem-cell research, obesity, gene therapy, alternative medicine, organ transplantation, mental health, and more.

PREFACE

It has been slightly more than a century since the first internal body structures were exposed to view in the intact human body. Wilhelm Roentgen's X-ray film revealing the bony structure of his wife's left hand ushered in a rush to apply the new technology for many things, some not so wise in retrospect. The risks of ionizing radiation exposure took over a decade to appreciate. However, the ability to see where a bone was fractured or the location of a bullet without surgery overcame the liabilities of the frivolous applications, and X-ray images greatly improved treatment. For millennia, practitioners of the healing arts had to deduce their patient's condition indirectly. Their methods ranged from consulting or casting out spirits, relying on the alignment of the planets, and identifying physical features of the patient, to divining imbalances among the four bodily humors (blood, phlegm, yellow bile, and black bile) or the four elements of the Earth (earth, air, fire, and water). Even when the understanding of disease had progressed from mysticism to physiology, societal and religious mores about the sanctity of the body prevented physicians from looking inside the body to find out what had happened, even after death.

Even with access to modern minimally invasive exploratory surgery, the holy grail of diagnostic medicine has been to see inside the intact human body. Transmission X-ray film radiograms were the standard for many decades, although X-ray scattering and overlapping features obscured details, and they were not so useful for soft tissues and organs. The utility of X-rays has been enhanced by a number of technologies, including the computer and the advent of two- and three-dimensional image reconstruction techniques borrowed from other fields. These processing technologies have been applied to other imaging modalities that employ different kinds of radiation to penetrate the skin and reveal functional as well as structural features of tissues, such as the brain, the heart, and the flow of blood in arteries and veins.

Medical Imaging follows the historical development of the technologies, many of which reached fruition only in the past twenty-five years or so, showing how advances in one area of science feed discovery and innovation in another. The workings of the technologies are collected in Section IIIB to avoid interruption of the story of their development. Physical principles are presented in more detail than most books on the topic for nonprofessionals in the field, without resorting to mathematics.

Although medical imaging is well established as a useful and often critical technology for better health care, it has not entirely avoided controversy. The lack of understanding in the past about the risks involved in exposure to ionizing radiation has been alleviated largely by studies that establish no-observable effect dosages and exposure limitations, to protect both the patient and the people operating the equipment.

Ethical concerns regarding use of medical imaging technologies as evidence in courts of law and in determining mental status, particularly for functional imaging of the brain, remain to be resolved. Medical imaging has even become embroiled in the controversy over abortion. Many states have passed legislation stipulating that before an abortion is conducted an ultrasound must be performed and the woman offered the opportunity to review the image "so that she may be fully informed" in her consent to the procedure. Abortion within the defined time limit is legal in the United States. Opponents view this as a form of coercion.

The major controversy surrounding high-tech imaging is the cost of the procedures and who is going to pay for them. Legislators, taxpayers, and health insurance companies are concerned that there is an economic incentive to overuse and abuse the technology. High-quality, high-technology equipment and trained professionals to operate it and interpret the output do not come cheaply nor are they accessible in less-economically advantaged areas or in developing countries. The tests can be invaluable, but to what extent are they being overused to cover physician liability and make up for less-skilled diagnosis?

ABBREVIATIONS

AACE	American Association of Clinical Endocrinologists
AEC	Atomic Energy Commission
AMIC	Access to Medical Imaging Coalition
BGO	bismuth-germanate
BOLD	blood oxygenation level-dependence
CDC	Centers for Disease Control
CNS	central nervous system
CSF	cerebrospinal fluid
CSSB	Committee Substitute for Senate Bill (Texas)
CT	computed tomography
DICOM	Digital Imaging and Communications in Medicine
DNA	deoxyribonucleic acid
DRA 2005	Deficit Reduction Act of 2005
EEG	electroencephalogram
EKG	electrocardiogram
EMG	electromyography
EPR	electron paramagnetic resonance
FCC	Federal Communications Commission
FDA	Food and Drug Administration
FDG	fluorodeoxyglucose
fMRI	fast MRI or functional MRI
FTC	Federal Trade Commission
GAO	Government Accountability Office

GPS	global positioning system
HIPAA	Health Insurance Portability and Accountability Act
MRI	magnetic resonance imaging
MRS	magnetic resonance spectroscopy
NMR	nuclear magnetic resonance
PACS	picture archiving and communications systems
PET	positron emission tomography
QALY	quality-adjusted life year
SPECT	single photon computed tomography
SQUID	super-conducting quantum interference devices
TENS	transcutaneous electric nerve stimulation

Units of Measure

cm	centimeter
eV	electron volt
GHz	gighertz − billion (10^9) cycles per second
Hz	hertz − cycles per second
kHz	kilohertz − thousand cycles per second
kV	kilovolts − thousand volts
keV	kiloelectron volts − thousand electron volts
MHz	megahertz − million (10^6) cycles per second
mm	millimeter
mV	millivolt
μm	micrometer

PART I

History and Scientific Background of Medical Imaging

CHAPTER 1

Before the Light—History of Looking Inside the Human Body

Modern medicine is a curious and sometimes uneasy alliance of the art of observation with technology. Diagnosis requires a blending of objective scientific tests with the patient's medical history and subjective impressions obtained during a physician's physical exam. Various diagnostic tests such as blood chemistries measure glucose, sodium and potassium, cholesterol and triglycerides, and monitor overall organ function as well as respiration rates, heartbeat, and body temperature. Technologies that are the subject of this book can image internal structures and activities within organs. They permit the physician to monitor the internal workings of the intact body at a level of detail unimagined a little more than a hundred years ago. Clinical observation of the patient during an exam feeds the subjective intuition accumulated by a skilled diagnostic physician from similar cases she has seen to build a sensible story. Even with all of the testing and accumulated clinical knowledge, in some situations, a physician still has to play a hunch to decide what is ailing a patient and how to treat him. This has been the experience throughout much of recorded history shared by those who have cared for the ill and the injured. Although this process seems decidedly unscientific and imprecise, the more relevant information the physician has at her disposal, the more accurate her diagnosis and therapeutic intervention can be.

Medical imaging technology was born in the winter of 1895 when a mysterious faint green glow tickled the curiosity of German physicist Wilhelm Roentgen as he hunched over a buzzing glass globe in his darkened wintry laboratory. His discovery of a light like no other fueled a popular curiosity that spread with phenomenal rapidity. Physicians immediately recognized the medical applications of X-rays. No other technology has ever been so enthusiastically adopted so soon after its demonstration. The race to see inside the intact human body was on. In the wake of X-ray radiography, a variety of imaging technologies based on other energy modalities were developed by physicists and engineers in collaboration with physicians. Each modality provided a unique perspective on the human body and its function. Imaging of the internal structures of the intact human body is now integral to standard diagnostic medical practice. At the time of the discovery of X-rays, seeing inside the human body was radical, even offensive to many people's sense of propriety. By contrast, medical imaging is now so routine that not using these powerful technologies can be grounds for malpractice lawsuits. For most of human history, though, the inside of the human body was a mystery.

DEVELOPMENT OF "INTERNAL" MEDICINE

Before the discovery of X-rays, not only could physicians not see into the human body, they were forbidden by their societies and religious strictures from doing anything other than observing and probing from the outside. These prohibitions were unanimous across different cultures, attesting to the reverence in which the human body was held. Many of these attitudes came from ignorance of the causes of disease and from superstition. At the time, such rules made sense within the local culture. If control of life by mystery and disease was divinely ordained, then disturbing the gods was dangerous, or at least heretical. There was plenty of opportunity to observe the inner workings of food animals, but humans were considered superior beings and therefore believed to be constructed differently. There was also ample opportunity to observe internal human anatomy—people were not averse to killing each other. They did so with great regularity, but warriors fighting in battle were one thing, whereas people, particularly sick people, were something else.

THE NATURE OF DISEASE

In addition to ignorance of human anatomy, notions of how the body functioned were poorly developed. Mysterious forces were called on to explain life and, its opposite, death. Without an understanding of how the body functioned, which we now call physiology, it is not surprising that concepts of illness tended to the mystical. People believed that disease was caused by evil spirits sent by the gods as punishment for not following some proscribed ritual. Opening a dead body was sure to attract the vengeance of the spirits. Superstition and magical explanations accounted for any phenomena that were not understood. According to the Hebrew scholar Rosner, the Jews believed "Only God could heal sickness" (Rosner 1977, p. 7). Some foreigners calling themselves *rofe* (healer) treated the ill. They were tolerated because they were useful, but were looked down on by the rest of society. Instead of treatment, the Jews focused on preventive medicine by stressing physical and mental hygiene. This was the rationale for some of the prohibitions and ritualizing of behavior such as prohibiting seafood and pork in a time of primitive food preservation methods.

Major civilizations evolved their own medical tradition. India was highly regarded for its highly developed surgical skills and tools. It also produced a vast compendia of medicinal knowledge freely mixed with religious philosophy and superstition. Many thought that diagnosis and the prospects for a patient's improved health were influenced by omens such as who the physician passed on his way to visit the patient. Little connection was made to what was happening to the body as a result of disease. The role of the internal organs in proper body function was not understood. This is readily explained as anatomy lessons were not easy to get. Ayurvedic writings of the fourth century A.D., noted that according to religious law, after a person's death the organs had to be put into a bag and allowed to rot in a river for seven days so that they could be dissected without having to use a knife. Much of the internal structure of the human body would not survive such treatment. The rise of Buddhism in the fourth century led to the decline of Indian surgical skills.

In China, anatomy was not investigated because Confucius taught that the body was sacred and should not be touched in death. Instead, Chinese medicine developed in other directions, producing a strong herbal medicine tradition. Immunization against smallpox was practiced in China long before being rediscovered by Western medicine in the seventeenth century.

THE RISE OF OBSERVATIONAL MEDICINE

The cooperation forged between the fiercely independent Greek city-states to resist invasion by Persia in the fifth century B.C. had a fortunate impact on Greek culture that advanced Western medicine. Greek medical tradition freely incorporated scientific notions about the body from Egypt, Mesopotamia, and Asia while playing down philosophical and religious dogma. A questioning attitude and tolerance for disagreement and discussion stimulated scholarship and prized the accumulation of new knowledge. The Greeks were great observers of many things, although much of their observation of the body was from the outside. Anatomical studies were not routine, but dissections of criminals or abandoned children were not ruled out. Clinical diagnosis involved the skillful use of the physician's ears, eyes, and hands when examining a patient, as well as common sense in interpreting the observations. Some of the descriptions and methods of gathering information are still used in the twenty-first century.

In the third century B.C., the Greek Ptolemaic emperors ruled Egypt. Alexandria, founded by Alexander the Great on the fertile delta at the mouth of the Nile River, became the home of one of the first scientific institutes. For the first time, systematic study of human anatomy was practiced. Herophilus and Erasistrasis "laid open men while still alive, criminals out of the prisons of the king and while they were still breathing" (Scarborough 1976). Dissections were performed for the most part on the young and healthy, thus contributing little opportunity for the discovery of the cause of an illness. For many illnesses, there was little appreciation for the physical effect of the pathologic process on the body, much less its root cause. The prevailing belief remained that invisible humors and not dysfunctional body organs were the cause of illness. As Greek supremacy in the Mediterranean waned, Alexandria was seriously damaged by a series of invasions by rival powers, and the city lost its prominence as a scientific center. Superstition returned to dominate Egypt. Attitudes shifted from trying to understand what caused illness to simply finding ways to cure it.

The remnant of the once-flourishing study of human anatomy in Alexandria following its decline as a scientific center was a single human skeleton displayed to the many physicians who still came to the city. Among them was a young man from present-day Turkey by the name of Galen. Like many others, after his training Galen went to Rome. There he performed public animal dissections and became an authority on many aspects of medicine. Although he avoided human dissection and despised surgery, he made considerable progress in understanding how the body functions (physiology). His approach was unique for his time. He made experimental lesions in animals, cutting nerves, muscles, and tendons, and watched for the consequences. Most important, he tried to relate his observations in his animal experiments to what he saw in his patients to deduce what might be wrong. Sometimes he was misled by differences between human and animal anatomy or misinterpreted what he observed with animals and then applied this to his patients. Nevertheless, by his death in 200 A.D., Galen had published more than 400 books and had become and would remain the dominant authority in medicine for more than one thousand years.

The Arabs who conquered Alexandria in 640 A.D., finished the job started by earlier invaders and demolished the city's great library along with its medical texts. Although the Arabs continued to make great strides in clinical observation and the use of medicines, the Koran prohibited dissections. This stricture effectively halted the study of anatomy and slowed the search for the causes of disease in the parts of the world under Islamic influence.

The situation was not much better in the non-Islamic world for many years. To the west, the collapse of the western Roman Empire and the rise of warrior fiefdoms, and heightened religious fervor during the Dark Ages (476–1000 A.D.) stymied progress in medicine in Christian Europe for nearly one thousand years, with notable exceptions. Only during the later Middle Ages (1000–1450 A.D.) did the practice of public dissections begin again. After miraculously surviving a bout with the bubonic plague that killed nearly a quarter of the population of Europe, and disgusted with the ignorance of physicians, Emperor Frederick II (1215–1250) decreed in 1238 that public dissections should be held at the medical school in Salerno. No one was allowed to perform surgery without having studied anatomy for one year.

In 1335, as part of a bid to improve medical education, the Venetian government required all licensed medical practitioners to attend an annual course of anatomy that included human dissection. The demonstrations were carried out with solemn ritual. Often the body was that of an executed criminal and the event was sometimes held in a church, usually during the winter to slow the rotting of the body. The order of dissection also was set by the rate of decay. First, the lower abdomen with the digestive system and liver was examined, followed by the chest with lungs and heart, ending with the skull. Increased numbers of dissections paralleled the wave of intellectual creativity and practical accomplishment that swept through Europe profoundly changing social attitudes—the Renaissance.

A NEW SPIRIT OF INQUIRY

Not surprisingly, painters and sculptors showed the most interest in anatomy, especially those in Florence. Leonardo da Vinci (1452–1519), painter of the *Mona Lisa* and the *Last Supper*, designer of menacing war machines and the helicopter, is said to have produced his detailed anatomical drawings from a series of thirty human dissections that he performed. His anatomic contributions, produced mostly after 1506, were largely unappreciated by his contemporaries because the bulk of his 750 drawings were not published until the late eighteenth century. Every detail was important. He made cross-sections of limbs and bones to look at their internal construction, and was the first to use a magnifying glass in biological work to examine the finer aspects.

Unschooled in medicine, and knowing no Greek and little Latin, he never consulted Galen's classic anatomy that had been in use for more than twelve centuries until he was far ahead of his predecessor. Da Vinci was an example in which seeing a subject with fresh eyes and no learned bias to overcome was an advantage. He corrected many of the errors perpetuated in Galen's writings due to the Greek's overextrapolation from his animal dissections, although he left some mistakes unaltered. He was not only a painter, sculptor, and inventor but also an anatomist and physiologist. Da Vinci used the sculptor's wax casting technique to preserve the true structures of the inside of blood vessels and the fluid-filled ventricular spaces in the brain that collapse after death. His drawings of the internal structure of his cadavers were strikingly reminiscent of images of live patients produced 450 years later by X-ray **angiography** and encephalography.

Da Vinci wanted to know not only what the blood vessels looked like, but also how they carried blood. He first made a wax cast of the inside of the aorta, a major blood vessel coming from the heart. After cutting the tissue away from around the wax, he coated the wax with Plaster of Paris, still used in the twenty-first century for plaster casts on broken legs or arms, and let it harden. After melting out the waxen core, he blew a thin coating of molten glass into the heat-resistant plaster mold. When he carefully chipped away the plaster, he was left with a thin clear glass tube that reproduced the inside contours of the original aorta. He then performed a series of experiments, blowing fine grass seeds through the tube and observing the flow and eddying of the tiny seeds as they passed along the inside of the vessel.

By 1520, not just artists but medical men were beginning to perform more human dissections, taking to heart the original meaning of the word "autopsy"—that is, personal or observation by the self—rather than pronouncing from learned texts and following the route Galen was on. Anatomical works of increasing accuracy appeared, and William Harvey's experiments and description of blood circulating from the heart through the lungs and back through the heart to the rest of the body cleared up a final remaining Galenic misconception.

CHAPTER 2

The Relationship of the Human Body and Disease

By the middle of the seventeenth century, accurate human gross anatomy was becoming fairly well established. What remained unresolved was how disease processes affected the body to create illness in the living patient. The effects of a knife or gunshot wound or the trauma of a broken leg or a skull fracture were understandable physical damage. Less obvious were illnesses that were hidden under the skin, inside the body. Dissections generally were performed on young, healthy (except for perhaps acute trauma) bodies, so little information was provided about what was going on inside. Physicians were still working blind.

CAUSES OF DISEASE

Until the eighteenth century, many physicians believed that illness was the result of bodily imbalances caused by miasmas, invisible vapors arising from swamps or dirty, overcrowded cities. Philosophical disputes raged between the miasmic concept of mysterious influences and the more physical contagion theories in which contact with the sick transmitted disease. Both of these explanations were used to account for what we now call infectious diseases, bubonic plague, diphtheria, and typhus, whose causative germs would be discovered in the mid-nineteenth century. However, neither cause could explain illnesses that did not pass from person to person, like a heart attack or apoplexy. A few physicians studying human anatomy, mainly at Italian universities, suggested that somehow damage to body organs caused illness, and they proposed that the clinical signs and outcome for the patient were related to what was happening to the effected organs. They began to gradually accumulate evidence for this radical idea.

Giovanni Battista Morgagni (1682–1771) at the University of Padua in Italy used the results of more than seven hundred autopsies to trace the footprint of several diseases by the changes he found in body organs. He described damage to the heart in angina and found that apoplexy, which we know as stroke, was due to clots in the blood vessels of the brain rather than a brain disease. Physicians gradually realized that damage to tissues and organs of the body were the hallmarks of diseases, although this was usually not obvious if the affected organs were internal until after the death of the patient. The microscope, a cousin of the newly invented telescope, provided a closer look at disease-ravaged organs and tissues.

Around 1600, Dutch spectacle makers constructed the first crude microscope. Its magnifying powers were soon put to use by Malpighi, a professor of medicine in Pisa, Italy. He was able to discern the detailed structure of a frog lung in which individual blood cells could be seen coursing through minute capillaries surrounding sac-like alveoli where gases were exchanged. This new instrument revealed that tissues and organs were built up from small cell units that were further organized into structures such as bones, teeth, muscles, and nerves. Critics countered, much as they did for Galileo and his telescope, that the microscopists were studying optical artifacts caused by their imperfect glass lenses, not real objects. In 1826, the surgeon father of Joseph Lister (the popularizer of antiseptics) produced a microscope with high magnification and superior achromatic optics that laid all doubts about the tricks of light to rest. Thin slicing of samples (microtomy) and color staining with chemical dyes (histology) produced by the German chemical industry and making certain components easily visible were standard by the 1880s. Medicine now had new eyes that could see deeper and more clearly than the early anatomists.

THE SCIENTIFIC BASIS FOR DISEASE

The newly born science of histopathology established the cellular basis of the modern notions of disease. Chemistry was being applied to biology, which led to advances in knowledge about how the body functioned (physiology) and how medicinal agents had their effects (pharmacology). Still, as the end of the century approached, physicians lacked visual confirmation of explanations for a disease in the living patient.

Paul Ehrlich (1854–1915), who discovered the first chemotherapeutic drug effective against syphilis wrote wistfully: "The staining of the dead gives us only anatomical clarification of architectural tissues. . . . If one wants to know about their function, one has to stain the normal tissues in the height of their activity" (Ehrlich 1886). This proved to be a prescient remark.

Despite new insight into physiological processes and the recognition that certain alterations of those processes caused by disease were responsible for particular illnesses, physicians remained limited in how they could detect these changes. They relied entirely on a few simple tests—count the pulse, measure blood pressure, measure body temperature, press and tap the body, and listen to the heart and lung sounds. Beyond that, the clinical experience of the physician must tell him (nearly all physicians then were men) what to expect. Successful diagnosis, though, did not necessarily improve the situation for the patient. Even if they knew what was wrong, there was little they could do for their patients. Often the only resource the physician could offer beyond surgery was morphine to ease pain.

THE EMERGENCE OF TECHNOLOGY

Just as there were impediments throughout early history to learning about human anatomy and how the body worked, those seeking to understand how the inanimate world worked encountered difficulties of a similar nature. The explanations for why objects fell to the ground, how birds flew, why the sun rose and set in the sky every day, the causes of weather, or the substance of lightning were magical and superstitious. The Greeks, for all of their innovation of representative government and acceptance of the superiority of reason and logic, allowed themselves to be ruled by their philosophy. Searching for truth in logic replaced the search for facts. Aristotle's and Galen's proscriptions on nature and health greatly retarded acceptance of experimental science as a way of knowing about the world.

Religious doctrine during the Middle Ages continued to consider adherence to philosophical and theological dogma superior to observation, which slowed progress in understanding the workings of the natural world. Unlike dissections, observations of nature and experiments generally were not prohibited, although publishing or teaching concepts that did not conform to the ruling theological persuasion could run a scientist afoul of the authorities, as Kepler, Copernicus, and Galileo found out.

Chemistry and physics escaped from philosophical bondage during the eighteenth century, gradually relying more and more on observation. It took medicine nearly a hundred years longer to accept experimental science as a way of advancing knowledge. In the late seventeenth century, the ancient Greek philosopher Democritus' concept that all matter was composed of small indivisible building blocks he called atoms, rather than of ephemeral mixtures of spirits and humors, began to receive experimental support. Lavoisier, Dalton, Avagadro, and others found that these "atoms" were a convenient way of explaining chemical changes. Atoms existed as a limited number of different kinds, called elements, and they joined in specific ways to make compounds. Chemists could empirically determine what combinations were allowed and in what proportion the combinations occurred, but they did not know why they formed. Physicists struggled to understand and explain the forces that governed the combinations and how they related to forces that shaped and moved the world.

Even before the natural forces were completely understood, they were rushed into harness to work for humankind. Michael Faraday described the connection between electricity and magnetism. Thanks to the inventive genius of Thomas Edison and others, the mysterious force of electricity gave rise to the telephone, the telegraph, the lightbulb, motion pictures, the electric trolley car, and countless other conveniences. People looked forward to the magical inventions coming out of the discoveries. Developments spawned by the industrial revolution, for all of their social consequences, allowed humankind for the first time to triumph over and control nature. Great ships powered by steam plied the oceans, and the steam-driven railroads tied the vast American continent together and connected the cities of Europe. The possibilities seemed endless.

Scientists were rapidly explaining the mysteries of everyday life in the latter part of the nineteenth and early twentieth centuries. A. A. Michelson, who would later win a Nobel Prize for his work on the physics of light, was moved to remark,

> The more fundamental laws and facts of physical science have all been discovered, and these are now so firmly established, that the possibility of their ever being supplanted in consequence of new discoveries is exceedingly remote. Our future discoveries must be looked for in the sixth place of decimal.

Such proclamations are issued periodically, even today, although history shows that new discoveries are always just over the horizon.

Having formulated the principles governing electricity, which provided the basis for the amazing inventions that became part of everyday life, physicists tried to explain the causes of the electrical effects. Experimentalists probed the smallest bits of matter for the answers. There were hints of even smaller components within atoms. Experiments were beginning to uncover and explain the most profound principles of nature. What the physicists found would improve the quality of life for millions, including developments leading to medical imaging technologies. Only later would they learn that their discoveries would also threaten a holocaust by releasing the energy from within the nucleus of the atom.

THE CONVERGENCE OF MEDICINE AND TECHNOLOGY—MEDICAL IMAGING

Near the end of the nineteenth century, the streams of progress in medical understanding and the growth of technology in harnessing the fundamental forces of nature were beginning to converge. They never were very far away from each other, largely because the scientific community was small and broadly interested in all fields of science. Physicians were often chemists or physicists in their spare time, and they often wrote to one another to discuss their latest discoveries.

Medicine had made enormous strides by the end of the nineteenth century in recognizing that the breakdown of the function of tissues and organs was the cause of disease. If physicians were able to determine what was wrong before the damage became severe, surgery under anesthesia provided some options for treatment. A limited number of medicines, mostly opiates for pain or weakly potent herbal remedies, were available. Chemotherapy was in its infancy, and the breakthrough of antibiotics was still in the future. Physicians and surgeons remained handicapped by not being able to see ahead of time the damage and potential complications caused by a disease. Within the short space of a year, near the very end of the nineteenth century, this situation changed as the result of a totally unanticipated discovery by an unknown but curious and observant physicist.

CHAPTER 3

First Light—The Discovery of X-Rays

On November 8, 1895, fifty-year-old Wilhelm Conrad Roentgen impatiently waited in his laboratory in the University of Wurzburg's Institute of Physics for the winter darkness so that he could get a series of experiments started before suppertime. He was fascinated with the newly described **cathode** rays generated by a Crookes tube, an oblong glass globe into which two wire electrodes had been sealed and from which the air had been removed. The cathode rays, later discovered to be **electrons**, produced a bright green glow on the inside wall of the tube. A colleague of his had found that a specially coated screen would also glow faintly when placed within three inches or so of the tube. Roentgen, an avid photographer, wanted to record this event.

Roentgen covered the Crookes tube with black cardboard to better see the dim, cathode ray–induced fluorescent glow on the screen in front of him and charged the electrodes. A little bit of the glow escaping from one end of the tube let him know that he was producing cathode rays. As he methodically tested the ability of thin sheets of paper, leather, glass, and metal to block the rays, Roentgen caught a faint gleam out of the corner of his eye. It was a faintly glowing letter "A," apparently written by a student on a piece of cardboard with a finger dipped in liquid barium platinocyanide used to coat viewing screens, lying on a chair a few feet away. He turned off the Crookes tube and the glow disappeared. It reappeared when he reenergized the tube. Neither cathode rays nor any other known rays could travel that far, so this was either some unknown form of energy or an artifact. Greatly excited, Roentgen continued to study his new phenomenon. Late in the evening, he went upstairs to his family apartment for dinner but sat silently distracted through the meal and then rushed back to his laboratory. He later wrote in his laboratory notebook, "I have discovered something interesting, but I do not know whether or not my observations are correct" (Glasser 1945).

Distrustful of his observations, Roentgen said nothing about his discovery to his assistants, and spent the next seven weeks characterizing and photographing the effects of the new rays on any kind of material he could lay his hands on. Thick books, wood, glass, rubber, tinfoil, all failed to stop this invisible light, which he called X-rays because they were mysterious. To his delight, the X-rays exposed photographic plates. Objects in a closed wooden box appeared on the photographic plate as if the box was not there. When he held his hand in front of the beam, the bones appeared in shadowy detail on a fluorescent screen.

On December 22, 1895, Roentgen brought his wife, Bertha, into the laboratory. She was the first person with whom he shared his discovery. He asked her to lay her hand on a photographic plate and charged the Crookes tube. The developed plate revealed the bones of her hand with her wedding ring suspended eerily around her finger. Immediately after Christmas, Roentgen sent copies of this picture and a manuscript detailing his discovery to the Wurtzburg Physical-Medical Society. The paper was published in the December 28 issue of 1895. By New Year's Day, he sent reprints of the article and copies of the photographic plate of Frau Roentgen's hand to several physics colleagues, one of whom passed the findings on to the press.

On January 5, 1896, the major European newspapers published the discovery, and within a week, articles on X-rays appeared in the leading medical journals in England, France, Germany, Italy, and the United States. During the succeeding months, numerous reports replicating Roentgen's findings appeared. Even in the days before mass media, within a year more than one thousand articles and forty-nine books were published on the X-ray phenomenon. A number of prominent physicists sheepishly realized that they too had encountered the effects of X-rays but had not been as observant or as persistent as Roentgen. No scientific discovery, before or since, has been as rapidly published and accepted by the public as were X-rays.

BENCHSIDE TO BEDSIDE IN RECORD TIME

The power and novelty of this new invisible light were embraced immediately by the world. It was another example of humankind's triumph over nature alongside the telegraph, the telephone, motion pictures, and the lightbulb. During the nineteenth century, technological advancements were hailed as progress with little thought as to the consequences. To his horror, Roentgen's discovery made him a celebrity. The rays were named **Roentgen rays** in his honor. He published just two more papers, in 1896 and 1897, on the properties of X-rays and then left the field forever. Roentgen was awarded the first Nobel Prize in Physics in 1901 for his discovery of X-rays. He donated the prize money to the University of Wurzburg.

The new rays were an instant sensation. Barely a month after Roentgen's paper, X-rays were used for the first time in a court of law in Canada to convict an assailant for shooting a man in a barroom brawl. The bullet was located in an X-ray radiograph after surgeons were unable to find it. Several months later, X-ray radiographs were introduced as evidence in a case of medical misdiagnosis in Denver, Colorado. Between 1896 and 1901, some eight thousand X-ray pictures were taken at Massachusetts General Hospital on three thousand patients.

Thomas Edison, America's renowned inventor, reportedly began construction on a darkroom to improve on the X-ray apparatus within hours of hearing of Roentgen's discovery. Edison's industrial-style laboratory in West Orange, New Jersey, replaced the platinum electrodes with aluminum and fashioned a thinner glass wall for the Crookes tube to increase the X-ray output. His assistants tested more than 8,500 substances in three months to find calcium tungstate, which glowed more brightly and produced crisper shadow images than Roentgen's screens. He quickly arranged for a nearby company to manufacture screens coated with the new agent. He also designed the fluoroscopic device used by Roentgen in his later studies. Edison produced complete X-ray kits, including power supplies, X-ray generating tubes, and his new **fluoroscope** for viewing the image. One of the first to contribute to the commercial use of X-ray devices, Edison was also one of the first to abandon working on them. He noticed a reddening around his eyes from using the fluoroscope, and one of his technicians lost fingers and eventually a hand from burns received from testing X-ray tubes.

Dentists rapidly took up the X-ray banner. By 1896, British dentists were routinely using X-rays to locate cavities. Tooth enamel absorbed X-rays better than bone, allowing dentists to check the formation and straightness of teeth, which they could see, even when buried in the bone of the jaw.

Medical uses dominated the early applications of X-rays and the equipment built to generate them. The Crookes tube produced X-rays as a by-product of a beam of electrons then known as cathode rays striking a metal **anode**. Since the human body was relatively transparent to X-rays, this weak source of X-rays was enough for early use. Trial-and-error experimentation produced powerful beams of X-rays even though workers did not know what X-rays were or understand how they were produced for almost fifteen years after their discovery. Once high power X-ray tubes were available, they were used in manufacturing to look for such things as bubbles inside metal castings or cracks in welds between two pieces of metal.

WARTIME SERVICE

X-rays were immediately pressed into medical service during the Spanish-American War in 1898, with Thomas Edison contributing a number of units designed for operation in the field. They proved excellent for assisting surgeons who could confidently find bullets and shrapnel, and align broken bones of wounded soldiers. They also showed that a crack in a small bone of the foot from prolonged marching caused the painful *pied forcé*, a nagging foot injury of infantry soldiers. These successes helped persuade conservative physicians that X-rays were more than a curiosity and could help them diagnose their patients.

By the time the hostilities of World War I broke out in August 1914, the high vacuum X-ray tube had been invented by General Electric engineer William Coolidge. It provided a consistent, high-intensity, focused source of X-rays, replacing the fragile and finicky Crookes gas tube. X-ray radiography helped save many lives and reduced the suffering of the wounded by showing the surgeon their internal injuries before he operated. Marie Curie, the discoverer of radium, trained female X-ray technicians and with the help of her seventeen-year-old daughter Irène who would one day win her own Nobel Prize, she outfitted touring cars as mobile X-ray laboratories at her own expense to aid the war effort. When the United States entered the war in April 1917, hundreds of the new **Coolidge tubes** (or C-tubes) were deployed to field hospitals, including a unit that could be wheeled from bed to bed in a ward for those patients too badly injured to be moved.

CARNIVAL SIDESHOW—THE CURIOUS SIDE OF X-RAYS

Roentgen's X-rays ignited a social craze unlike any other discovery. Within weeks of the publication of his paper, X-rays were suddenly everywhere. Building an X-ray device was simple for anyone with any mechanical and electrical aptitude. Coin-operated X-ray machines would give a view of the bones in the hand of the curious. Bloomingdale's department store gave demonstrations of X-rays alternating with showings of the newly introduced motion pictures. X-ray Boy's Clubs sprang up around the United States. X-ray booths were set up in shoe stores so patrons could view how their new shoes fit their feet. Devices such as the Foot-O-Scope and their glowing screens remained a fixture in shoe stores for more than forty years.

The power of X-rays to make the invisible visible fired the imagination of writers. H. G. Wells's scientist hero in *The Invisible Man* (1897) discovered mysterious rays that rendered him invisible, except for right after he had eaten a meal when the food was visible in his stomach until it was absorbed. Invading Martians armed with death rays destroyed Earthlings and their military in his *The War of the Worlds* (1898). Superman's X-ray vision let him see through walls, although the reality is that X-rays pass through most objects and are not reflected back to produce an image even if eyes could focus on or were sensitive to X-rays.

At the turn of the twentieth century, some people were uncomfortable with the revealing powers of X-rays. They felt that the last barrier of privacy, a person's skin, had been taken away. Others felt that it was immoral for internal organs to be on display, echoing the taboos of earlier centuries against looking inside the human body. Many people were frightened. Frau Roentgen reportedly thought she was seeing her own death when she saw the ghostly image of the bones of her hand. As X-rays proved their value in accurate diagnosis and improved the quality of care in medicine and dentistry, public discomfort with perceptions of body image evaporated. In the twenty-first century, failure to properly use modern X-rays or other medical imaging methods for diagnosis and planning of therapy is considered malpractice.

Progress Can Kill—The Dangers of Overexposure

The discovery of X-rays was one of the few discoveries in the modern era of physics that was completely unexpected. X-rays were observed experimentally before there was a theory to explain them. Their kinship with visible light as another form of **electromagnetic radiation** was finally recognized by von Laue and associates in 1912, after Ernest Rutherford's model of the atom provided an explanation for the production of X-rays. These studies revealed the high energy present in X-rays. The medical reports, as early as 1905, of delayed reaction to heavy doses of X-rays and the sores and cancers afflicting early radiographers now made some sense. Before X-rays, people were used to thinking about direct and immediate consequences of events. A burn from a hot stove raises a blister within minutes. By contrast, the effects of an X-ray burn may show up weeks or months after exposure. Effects on fertility or cancers might appear up to twenty years later. No wonder few patients or physicians made the connection between cause and effect of X-rays.

To further confuse the issue, exposure to high doses of X-rays was not entirely negative. There were also some desirable effects. Acne sores healed, tumors shrank, and unsightly birthmarks faded. In hindsight, overzealous X-ray treatments for some of these conditions may have caused more problems than they helped, but any increase in cancers would have been so long after the exposure, no one would have made the connection. By the 1930s, radiologists and manufacturers finally agreed on a standard of tolerable radiation exposure that defined a level to which a patient or radiation worker could be exposed with a low probability of consequences. As better measures of the effects of X-rays and other forms of radiation were developed, this arbitrary dosage was lowered.

Most of the early exposure, and thus many of the effects of X-rays, were found among the people who worked with the instruments that generated them—that is, radiologists, X-ray technicians, and manufacturers and testers of the X-ray generating tubes. Nearly all of the early radiographers lost fingers, hands, and arms, often suffering great pain. They had fewer children and experienced a larger proportion of malformed infants. Most considered these tragedies the price of being in the forefront of their occupation and chose to continue. Many became martyrs to their craft, eventually dying from cancer or infection resulting from radiation-induced sores that refused to heal in the time before antibiotics. Elizabeth Fleischman, a pioneering radiographer renowned for her detailed X-ray photographs, lost an arm, and died of cancer in 1905. Marie Curie died of leukemia in 1934 at age sixty-seven, a result of the accumulated effect of exposure to the rays emitted by the radium she handled with little thought for her own safety. The dangers of overexposure to high-energy radiation were beginning to be realized around the time of her death.

Imaging with X-rays shattered both the physical and psychological barrier of the skin. It was finally possible to see within the intact living human body. What physicians saw enabled them to diagnose conditions more rapidly and more accurately, thus allowing them to save many lives. X-rays opened the way for discovery of other kinds of medical imaging. People began to think about what other sorts of energy forms could penetrate the skin to reveal what was inside. Now there was a real need to see inside, and patients were demanding that this need be met.

RADIATION AND IMAGING—GETTING THE PICTURE

The discovery that X-rays could reveal the inner structures of the body through the skin triggered a revolution in technology and started people thinking about how to improve the quality of the blurry images and to increase the amount of detail that could be discerned. A bullet or a bobby pin were obvious to any observer, but physicians wanted to know more about internal organs that were deeper in the body and what they looked like in disease and in health. Tissues other than bone were hard to see clearly because their density was similar to the surrounding water. Air in the lungs created sufficient contrast to reveal tissue structure, but lungs were an exception. It still required experience to interpret the shadows and hazy shapes. Lung damage from tuberculosis infection showed up as dark spots and splotches.

Photographic emulsions, a thin layer of radiation-sensitive chemical coated onto glass plates or now a flexible plastic backing film, were the medium used to record the first X-ray pictures and remain the least expensive and most popular medium in the twenty-first century. X-ray imaging operates by recording the intensity of a beam of X-rays that passes through the subject to a detector, usually film, on the opposite side. The X-ray beam is left on until enough X-rays have passed through the subject to expose the film sufficiently for a negative or inverse image to form—clear (unexposed) where the X-rays are blocked by something like bone and dark where the X-rays were only weakly absorbed by soft tissue or water. Unlike a camera, there is no lens, only a **collimator** tube that passes only X-rays moving parallel to the long axis of the tube. This improves the sharpness of the image because all of the X-rays are traveling in the same direction, carrying information about the subject directly in their path. X-rays traveling at an angle do not carry useful information and just fog the film. Because of their high energy and thus short **wavelength**, X-rays are not bent or focused readily by lenses such as those used for visible light. They can be managed by mirrors and by **grazing-angle reflection** from certain kinds of crystals that have been applied in the design of space X-ray telescopes or X-ray **crystallography** devices used to determine molecular structures. However, this has not been practical for medical imaging.

X-rays pass through the body and produce a shadow image on photographic film or some other detector of X-rays on the other side. Our brain is used to interpreting visible wavelengths of light reflected back from an object to our eyes as an image. Radiologists have to learn how to read these negative images. If our eyes could detect X-rays (assuming they were somehow protected from radiation damage) objects that either absorbed or scattered those X-rays would appear solid to us and would look dark. If we substituted our eyes with a piece of film, absorption of the X-rays would leave that area on the film unexposed and the processed film would be clear or light in that area. This shadow X-ray image is like a black-and-white photographic negative in which areas of the image where light was absorbed are clear and where light exposed the film are dark. For twenty-first-century digital camera generation, an X-ray film image looks like a digital image in which light and dark are inverted as a special effect.

The biggest problem in obtaining sharp film X-ray images was film exposure due to stray radiation that either excited within tissue molecules by the highly energetic X-rays or scattered off of areas of differing tissue density. This secondary radiation was emitted in all directions. Also, like other forms of light, X-rays slightly deviate (refract) from a straight-line path when they pass through areas of different density (e.g., bone, fat, water, cartilage, muscle). Recently, this refraction has been harnessed to reveal detail in weakly contrasted soft tissue (see Chapter 5 on mammography). A certain fraction of the radiation reflects off of each interface of different density. The result at the level of the recording device is that a significant amount of secondary or scattered X-ray intensity is unrelated to the image information. This degrades image sharpness by fogging the film, producing the effect of looking at a piece of art through a heavily smudged pair of glasses.

In 1913, a German physician, Gustav Bucky, devised a simple method of collimating the X-rays by inserting one grid of thin X-ray-absorbing strips between the patient and the X-ray tube and another below the patient just above the film recording the transmitted X-rays. The strips allowed X-rays to pass through the holes in the grid but blocked any that were going sideways, greatly reducing the scattering and drastically improving image quality. An American in Chicago, Hollis Potter, further improved the invention in 1915 by moving the grids slightly during the exposure, smearing out the annoying Bucky grid lines in the image. Collimating the X-rays had the additional benefit of allowing larger images than the 4×5 inch glass plates, which were a compromise with the increased scattering of larger formats, and speeding the transition from the delicate glass plates to the familiar plastic (cellulose ester)-backed 14×17 inch X-ray films.

IN THE SHADOW OF X-RAYS—CONTRAST AGENTS

Foreign metal objects were easy to pick up in X-ray images. However, tissues other than bone were made up primarily of hydrogen, carbon, nitrogen, and oxygen. These "light elements" contain low numbers of protons and neutrons and consequently interact weakly with X-rays. While this allows X-rays to readily penetrate the body to reveal internal structures, it also makes most soft tissues nearly invisible on X-rays. As discussed in later chapters on magnetic resonance imaging and ultrasound, this deficiency stimulated the search for other technologies that could produce images of soft tissues. Imagers began to try nonionizing forms of radiation to exploit other "windows" into the intact body.

Still, X-rays did certain things very well, so specialists tried changing some of the imaging conditions to enhance features that they wanted to observe. To accentuate certain details or merge aspects of an image, film photographers use different colored filters to change the characteristics of the light reaching the film. This results in changes in the differences, the contrast, between elements of the image, making certain things easier to see. Anode X-ray generator composition and special metal filters that only allowed X-rays of specific moderate energies through improved some soft tissue details.

A more successful approach involved altering the X-ray density of a target organ or tissue in a systematic way. Histological stains had been developed in the early nineteenth century to provide contrasting color to what was mostly crystal-clear tissue slices prepared for light microscopy. Physicians observed that air in the lungs transmitted X-rays significantly differently than watery tissue or bone. Since the density of air is less than water, X-rays are absorbed less by the air, resulting in more X-rays reaching and darkening the film in that part of the image. In 1918, sterile air injected into the ventricles of the brain, a notoriously difficult tissue from which to obtain satisfactory X-ray images, displaced the **cerebrospinal fluid** (CSF) normally present there strikingly delineating those cavities with dark shadows. A similar technique, dubbed air **myelinography**, was introduced in 1921 to image the nerve channel in the spinal column.

The air would eventually be absorbed and the ventricles refilled with CSF, but this was an uncomfortable procedure for the patient.

A lower-density medium for contrast was not the answer for all imaging applications. Air injected into a blood vessel would block blood flow resulting in an **embolism**. An alternative strategy was to introduce materials with higher density than water. Elements with high **atomic number** (high number of protons and neutrons), such as the calcium in bones, interact strongly with X-rays and show up well in X-ray radiograms. The first **arteriogram**, visualization of blood vessels, employed the high atomic number water-soluble material salt, strontium (atomic number 38) bromide. Higher contrast was obtained in 1931 with Thorotrast, made with thorium (atomic number 90), which had a higher **atomic number** than strontium, but the radioactivity of this element was a problem as the dangers of exposure to radioactivity were beginning to be appreciated. A variety of agents for different purposes were tested, including bismuth or barium salts, which are still used in the twenty-first century to coat the gastrointestinal tract (barium swallow) to look for lesions of various types. Less toxic materials that incorporated iodine into water-
soluble organic molecules also proved useful.

Just as histological stains could be directed to specific targets by careful selection of the stain's chemical structure, it is possible to similarly direct X-ray **contrast agents** incorporating high atomic number elements to specific targets to highlight particular conditions. A similar strategy is used to target **radiopharmaceuticals** in nuclear imaging (see SPECT and PET in Chapter 7). Contrast agents, with and without specific targeting, are useful for many of the medical imaging modalities. The molecular nature of a contrast agent depends on the physical nature of the interaction of the imaging radiation with the tissue. The use of contrast agents will be described for each of the modalities.

CHAPTER 4

The Body in Motion—Fluoroscopy

Wilhelm Roentgen's discovery was the astute observation of a glint of green **fluorescence**, and his original experiments showed that this new kind of light, which he called X-rays, was not the well-known cathode rays generated by the Crookes tube. It was quick and easy, but the image on the barium platinocyanide–coated plate was fuzzy and dim. Besides, as a scientist, he needed to make a permanent record that he could show others. Photographic emulsions were sensitive to the new rays. The famous picture of Frau Roentgen's hand with her wedding ring floating eerily on the X-ray lucent flesh required a fifteen-minute exposure with his weak source. As the control and intensity of X-ray sources improved with the advent of the Coolidge tube, exposure times decreased, but motion remained an anathema for high-quality static imaging for which the fine details of anatomical structure were important. Movement due to heart activity or breathing during X-ray exposure caused blurring. A great deal of effort has gone into minimizing the effects of motion on the images.

The motion problem for static high-resolution images contained a silver lining. Depending on the target, the motion of organs and tissues was itself of interest to physicians. Even if the image was blurry, it was clear enough to determine how well the organ was functioning. With a fluorescent screen, the motion could be followed in real time. X-rays could be used to observe the function of internal organs. A tissue or organ could sometimes look completely anatomically normal over the interval of an X-ray exposure, yet be causing a medical condition because it was not operating properly. Examples of this include the lungs, heart cycle, the stomach and intestinal tract, and knee and ankle joints. Real-time observation with X-rays was possible using fluorescent screens. Thomas Edison's brighter calcium tungstate screens helped, but images were dim and required radiologists using fluorography to spend long periods of time in the dark until their eyes regained sufficient sensitivity to see details in the images. Kymography of heart motion was captured by recording the image on the fluorescent screen by moving a strip of film past a slit. This principle was reminiscent of Edison's motion pictures, but the images were crude.

To obtain a useable image, some means of increasing the brightness and sharpness was needed. The fluorescent screens, even the ones Edison developed, had to be used in near total darkness, and the radiographer's eyes needed to be dark-adapted. There were limitations on the intensity of X-rays both for image quality and for patient safety. A fundamentally different way to increase the light output stimulated by X-rays interacting with a fluorescent screen was needed. Technology soon came to the rescue. Attempts at a creating a device that would amplify the light in an image began to succeed as television was developed in the 1940s. From that point, coupling television technology with intensifying screens was inevitable. Russell Morgan at Johns Hopkins University coupled the two in 1948 and demonstrated the utility. A year later, Richard Chamberlain and Sam Seal at RCA Victor combined a television videocon tube with an intensifier screen that not only produced an amplification of the light image that was fifty thousand times greater, but the refresh rate was sufficiently rapid that motion of organs during coughing, swallowing, and cardiac motion could be observed. Eventually, fluorescent screens were replaced by position-sensitive crystals and semiconductor materials from which X-rays dislodged electrons that were accelerated by a high voltage through a cascade of steps producing a detectable current. The development of this technology and the improvements that followed ushered in a new era in radiology. Not only could function be observed, but arterial and cardiac surgery was made safer and less invasive because catheterizations could be followed in real time as the devices were inserted and moved to their target. Angiography using X-ray-absorbing contrast agents to visualize the integrity of the blood vessels could detect blockages of vessels and guide the intravascular surgical instruments into position to repair the damage. The Nobel Prize in Medicine and Physiology was awarded in 1956 for the visualization of internal organs of the human body to André Cournaud, Werner Forssman, and Dickinson Richards.

CHAPTER 5

Breast Cancer Detection—Mammography

Perhaps one in nine American women will develop breast cancer during their lifetime. One hundred and eighty thousand new cases are reported each year. The good news is that when detected early, the five-year survival rate for breast cancer is around 90 percent. The emphasis is now on early detection, and the earlier the better. In the absence of a sensitive blood test and the limited sensitivity of detection of small deep tumors by manual palpation, physicians turned to imaging methods. X-ray imaging was able to visualize tumors in other tissues, but soft breast tissue presented a number of technical obstacles.

Early X-ray studies revealed almost no discernable internal structure in the soft tissue of the human breast. Screeners for tuberculosis could easily see the lung tissue with little interference from overlying breast tissue. Palpation by a physician was the only means of breast cancer detection. However, by X-ray, imaging tumors looked very much like normal breast tissue. In the early twentieth century, breast cancer was dealt with by radical mastectomy, surgical removal of the breast, any associated lymphatic system, and the underlying muscle. After the beneficial effects of X-rays on reducing tumor size were appreciated, mastectomy became somewhat less radical and was augmented with high-intensity X-ray treatments.

Radiologists kept trying to find some kind of signature of breast tumors. Albert Salomon's careful X-ray observations in three thousand mastectomy specimens in 1913 in Berlin frequently turned up small dark dots, later shown to be microcrystals of calcium, accumulating at the centers of the tumors. The reason for the crystals in breast tumors was not clear. They did not appear in most tumors in other tissues. Nevertheless, these X-ray absorbing microcrystals became an important diagnostic aid in the early detection of breast tumors as the technology was gradually improved to the point at which density differences between the tumor and normal breast tissue could be resolved. Salomon's studies were followed up in the 1930s by Jacob Gershon-Cohen at Jefferson Medical College in Philadelphia, but it was not until 1949 that Raul Leborgne identified calcium microcrystals in 30 percent of cancer cases.

Direct detection of breast tumors became possible after Charles Gros of Strasbourg, France, who was wrestling with the technical problems of obtaining useful images, developed a new breast compression method. This method produced a more uniform tissue thickness and improved the contrast in the image so that small differences in tissue density could be discerned. This was the key to locating early tumors. Specialized radiological equipment designed explicitly for **mammography** first hit the market in 1967. Xerox adapted their method of recording images on a selenium-sensitized aluminum plate to recording high-resolution, high-contrast X-ray mammograms. The competition stimulated the X-ray equipment manufacturers to further refine their technology. Switching anode materials from molybdenum to tungsten produced lower energy and therefore less penetrating X-rays that gave better soft tissue contrast. The reduced penetration of these weaker X-rays was compensated for by breast compression and increased detector sensitivity.

The potential for early detection and treatment provided by screening mammograms for breast cancer ignited considerable interest among health care professionals and in the general population. The highly publicized breast cancers of Betty Ford and Happy Rockefeller in 1974 further brought mammograms into the mainstream. The debate over the risk-benefit and the cost of yearly mammograms for women forty years and older still smolders in the twenty-first century. Even with improvements in equipment, studies found that radiologists reading mammograms missed 15 percent of cancers. Since the differences between normal breast and cancerous tissue are subtle, this is not surprising, but it needs to be addressed.

Computer-assisted reading of radiograms is reducing the number of false negatives. A major contribution to this effort came from an unlikely source. After its 1993 launch, the main mirror of the Hubble Space Telescope suffered from spherical aberration severe enough to jeopardize the mission. Software **algorithms** were developed to compensate for the spherical aberration, to discriminate cosmic ray-generated noise on the telescope camera and to pick out faint stars from the fuzzy background. Radiologist and pioneer in digital radiography Matthew Freedom at the Georgetown University Lombardi Cancer Institute took advantage of the algorithms, adapting them to his problem of picking out the tiny faint calcifications signaling early stage breast cancer from the tissue background.

DIFFRACTION-ENHANCED X-RAY IMAGING FOR SOFT TISSUE

The low density of breast tissue and the weak absorption of standard-energy X-rays as they pass through its intricate but weakly contrasting structure hamper detection of cancerous lesions. Lower-energy X-rays interact more strongly with the tissue, but even with the compression systems used to reduce the thickness of the imaged area, not enough X-rays under normal circumstances penetrate to the detector to produce a useful image. In 1995, scientists at the National Synchrotron Light Source at Brookhaven National Lab took advantage of a property of X-rays common to light and all forms of electromagnetic radiation that allowed them to enhance very small contrast differences in a sample volume (Chapman et al. 1997).

There are three types of interaction of electromagnetic radiation, which includes X-rays, with a medium through which they pass: absorption, refraction, and scattering. Absorption of X-rays is the basis for traditional X-ray radiography in which contrast arises from the differential absorption of the radiation by tissue components. The new technique focuses instead on refraction. It operates by measuring the slight changes in direction of X-rays caused by bending of their path as they pass through areas of different density, also called refractive index. The scattering of X-rays as they pass through tissue that causes so much difficulty with image fuzziness in standard radiography is over a much greater angle and they can be filtered out without losing the refraction information. When a beam passes through, the subject is compared with a portion of the beam that did not pass through the subject, and the difference highlights boundaries of the areas where the X-rays were bent, yielding an improvement of more than tenfold in contrast. The data can be separated into an absorption image and a refraction image, and three-dimensional images can be produced as well (Dilmanian et al. 2000).

Several other advantages of **diffraction** imaging over absorption imaging are that the size of the diffracting object does not matter until it reaches the dimensions of the X-ray wavelength nor does the energy of the X-rays. This is important because X-rays of sufficient energy to penetrate the tissue of interest can be used and the radiation dose can be quite drastically reduced, tenfold or more. This is of obvious benefit to the patient, particularly for diagnostic screening of breast cancer in which multiple scans are performed over a lifetime, by lowering the cumulative exposure.

A limiting factor to the development of this method for medical imaging is that it relies on a source of X-rays with a single or narrow range of energies (wavelengths). A silicon crystal is used to selectively diffract a narrow range of X-ray energies for scanning the subject. A similar crystal removes scattered radiation after it emerges from the subject. These manipulations are necessary to protect the quality of the image. Just as the refractive index of a prism separates white light into its component colors, an X-ray beam of multiple energies (wavelengths) would be spread similarly at the boundaries of different density, which would blur the image. An impediment to the routine application of this technology is the size and complexity of the equipment needed to produce a narrow range of X-ray wavelengths although compact sources are now in development (Parham et al. 2009).

CHAPTER 6

Three-Dimensional Imaging—The Development of Tomography

The vast majority of X-ray images taken in the twenty-first century, like a chest X-ray, dental X-rays, or a shot of a hand, are two-dimensional records on film of the absorbance of X-rays passing through a part of the body. This is sufficient, in many cases, to detect a tubercular lesion on the lung, a cavity in a tooth, or a break in a bone. The process is rapid and inexpensive. The images, however, are two-dimensional and indistinct because they contain absorption information and X-rays scattered from all of the tissue between the X-ray source and the film. Details of deeper lying structures are obscured by the haze, even to the trained eye of an experienced radiologist. Some structures hidden beneath strongly X-ray-absorbing bone cannot be imaged effectively. These deficiencies were realized early in the development of X-ray technology. The Bucky-Potter grid system reduced the amount of scattered radiation fogging the film, and moving the grids kept their shadow from registering on the film. Absorption that resulted from overlying features, such as organs, was unaffected by this strategy however. This interference continued to render the image indistinct, and strongly absorbing bone, such as the skull or ribs, completely obliterated the image of underlying structures. At least instrument makers were on the right track by removing image distortion caused by scattered radiation, but X-ray absorption from above and below the region of interest still obscured much important detail.

Mechanical systems such as one demonstrated in 1930 by Allesandro Vallebona used motion to isolate specific image information. The technique was called **tomography**, from the Greek *tomos* meaning section, slice, or cut. The slice was generated by synchronously moving the X-ray tube and the film around a common axis centered on the patient to purposely blur all image information from outside of that region. The technique was crude however, and it proved difficult to engineer the precise movement of the heavy mechanical equipment. A solution came from an unrelated source.

Various solutions to extracting two- or three-dimensional information from a series of one-dimensional projections have surfaced multiple times in different areas of science and engineering. Mechanical tomographic methods were appropriate for certain applications, but not for others. Fortunately, several investigators recognized that mathematical manipulation of the observational data could produce equivalent or even superior multidimensional output. Austrian mathematician Johann H. Radon was wrestling in 1917 with an astrophysical problem trying to reconstitute a three-dimensional image from a series of two-dimensional projections. Like Gregory Mendel's genetics observations on pea plants, Radon's published algorithms went unnoticed and then were lost.

In the 1950s, an astronomer, Ronald Bracewell, at Stanford University reconstructed solar-radio telescope images using mathematical Fourier transformation. He abandoned this approach and substituted less computationally intensive methods in the 1960s. The mathematical constructs were available, but computing resources (initially pencil and paper and finally early electronic computers) were inadequate, particularly for anything time-sensitive such as a medical application. Bracewell's methods, however, were buried in an Australian physics journal not read by physicians. Similar methods were applied in the 1960s by biologist Aaron Klug and colleagues to determine the three-dimensional structure of a tobacco mosaic virus, which was too small to see with a regular light microscope. Klug and colleagues manipulated images of the virus taken at different angles with a microscope that used a beam of electrons to produce highly magnified images. Still, these were relatively simple situations. No one was working with a three-dimensional subject with density differences as complex as the human body.

As was apparent with the discovery of X-rays, the same good idea occurs to many people when the time is right, but most do not realize it until after someone else brings it into the public eye. Multiple investigators with different backgrounds provided the experimental and mathematical impetus that lead to medical X-ray tomography. William Oldendorf was a neurologist with an engineering bent who wanted to spare his patients the painful injection of air used to highlight the ventricles of the brain. The dense bone of the skull seriously interfered with X-ray studies of the brain. He was not satisfied with the quality of X-ray images of brain tissue even when the bone had been removed.

Stimulated by talking with an engineer who had been hired to produce a device to detect intact but frost-bitten oranges, he came up with the notion of following up on mechanical tomography by setting up a narrow radiation beam and an electronic detector positioned 180 degrees apart and rotating the subject between them. By replacing the film with electronics, he could electronically filter out unwanted information. He went home and built a **test phantom**, a three-dimensional block of plastic mounted with a forest of iron nails, one steel nail, and a single aluminum nail that absorbed gamma rays and X-rays differently than the other nails. His scanner was a sixteen revolution per minute (rpm) record player turntable that in addition to rotating also could be moved in a straight line on a section of HO-scale model railroad track borrowed from his son's train set. He placed his phantom on this scanner between a fixed narrow beam of gamma rays emitted from a small lead-shielded radioactive source and his detector. This simple device addressed all of the fundamental concepts used in later computerized scanners except that there was no computer. Oldendorf was able to produce a two-dimensional image locating the aluminum nail among the iron nails in his phantom.

He obtained a patent in 1963 for his concept, but when he approached major X-ray manufacturers, he was told by one, "Even if it can be made to work as you suggest, we cannot imagine a significant market for such an expensive apparatus which would do nothing but make radiographic cross-sections of the head" (Oldendorf 1980). After this rebuff, Oldendorf abandoned imaging and spent the rest of his career studying the blood-brain barrier.

Alan Cormack, a physicist in South Africa, built a scanner similar to Oldendorf's in 1957 and devised a mathematical treatment called a line-integral method to analyze the intensity changes in the transmitted energy. In 1963, he moved to Tufts University in Boston and constructed a system that used a computer to perform the image **reconstructions**. He tried to interest a group of physicians at Massachusetts General Hospital who were using new **radioisotopes** produced by a **cyclotron** to investigate the differences between normal and malignant tissue in using his mathematical methods for emission scanning of radioisotopes in those tissues. They were not convinced that the technique would be useful, and Cormack drifted into a department chairmanship. It was ten years later before physicians saw the light and adopted his approach for **nuclear imaging** of radioisotopes.

The first cross-sectional image made by sending a beam of radiation through a living subject to detectors was published in 1966 by David Kuhl at the University of Pennsylvania. It was a sophisticated computerized device; however, it used gamma rays and could produce only a cross-sectional image, it was not a computerized scanner. Although all of the components were available, Kuhl was not focused on three-dimensional transmission imaging, but on emission imaging of an internal source of radiation (see Chapter 7 on SPECT and PET imaging).

The man who provided the connection between computational tomography theory and practical application was Godfrey Hounsfield, born in 1919, a bright and curious son of an English farmer, but a weak student who never attended university. He worked for a home-builder until World War II began. In 1939, Hounsfield was assigned to the communications section of the Royal Air Force. He did so well on the entrance exam that instead of taking the course, he was assigned to teach it and went on to distinguish himself doing research on the new top-secret radio detection and ranging (RADAR) technology.

After the war he joined EMI, the English Gramophone Company, which had an interest in transistors and computers. EMI's signature product, however, was musical recordings, which in the 1960s included groups such as the Beatles. Hounsfield was assigned to their central research laboratory where he was allowed to work on anything that was related in some way to their business, much like the Bell Telephone Research Laboratories in the United States. He began work on computers but soon took up the problem of pattern recognition, which dealt with information content of various kinds of signals. His experience with RADAR combined with the rapidly advancing computer technology lead him to the same conclusions as Oldendorf, Cormack, and Kuhl, which up to that point had failed to result in a practical application.

Hounsfield was fortunate to work for a director of research with a sense of vision. When EMI balked at funding the project on its own, his director, Len Broadway, sought partners with an interest in brain scans, including the Department of Health and Social Security and the neurosurgeon James Ambrose. Beginning in 1967, the joint venture between EMI and the Medical Research Council gave Hounsfield the resources to build prototype equipment. His first scans of a model brain (phantom) used gamma rays for simplicity, but it took nine days for the scan and two and a half hours for the computer processing. Switching to a more intense X-ray source cut the scan time down to nine hours, which was still impractical.

On October 1, 1971, Ambrose and Hounsfield performed the first clinical computed tomography (CT) imaging by scanning the head of a woman who had symptoms of a brain tumor. Data were acquired in one-degree increments over a total of four minutes. The data were stored on magnetic tape and sent across town to a computer to produce an image. A photograph of the computer monitor screen clearly revealed the tumor, which Ambrose successfully removed.

The response in the neuroradiology community to the first CT scan was reminiscent of the reaction to publication of Roentgen's X-ray film in 1896. EMI was soon producing scanners as fast as possible, and they established a U.S. operation in Reston, Virginia, home of the American Radiology College. Patients lined up in clinics as neurologists sought a three-dimensional view of the brain that greatly reduced the number of exploratory surgeries for an organ that previously had been almost inaccessible to imaging technology. Contrary to the projection of the medical equipment manufacturer who saw limited utility for tomographic scanning, instruments were soon designed that could image any portion of the body. The three-dimensional imaging allowed physicians to obtain clear pictures of organs and tissues that lay underneath bony structures, such as the ribs, that had been obscured on traditional X-ray films.

Modern CT scans can be done quickly. The data are acquired in a series of two-dimensional "slices" about 5 to 10 millimeters in thickness, depending on the part of the body being imaged. The X-ray generator moves in stepwise increments in a vertical circle around the subject, while the X-ray detectors directly opposite the generator record the absorption of the X-rays, which is related to the tissue density. The platform on which the subject is lying is moved ahead the distance of a slice thickness and the scanning process is repeated. The number of slices collected depends on the size of the area being imaged. The computer takes the data from each slice and calculates the X-ray absorption at each point where the X-ray beams coming from the many angles of the stepwise incremental exposures intersect. (Each point is a volume element called a **voxel**.) The absorbance calculated in Hounsfield units is then presented as a density on film, a paper printout, or computer screen for the radiologist to interpret.

Traditionally, the X-ray absorption data are presented as cross-sectional axial segments, but they are not limited to that projection. The computer can use the same data to calculate displays from additional perspectives,

sagittal (lengthwise side-to-side) or **coronal** (top to bottom like a layer cake), to make particular features stand out to the radiologist. Despite the total number of X-ray pictures taken, the amount of X-rays the subject is exposed to is only somewhat more than that required for a standard film X-ray series, because the sensitivity of modern detectors permits lower X-ray doses. Three-dimensional images can be computed from the two-dimensional slices to give the radiologist and surgeons a more anatomically realistic image of structures, although in practice, the slices provide enough information for a diagnosis.

Modifications to this general procedure are made when particular body features are of interest. Faster acquisition of sectional data with some tradeoff of resolution is obtained by **spiral CT** scanning where the area of interest is continuously moved through the rotating X-ray beam. By triggering data collection off of physiological events, such as breathing or the heartbeat, motion artifacts can be removed. This technique also can be used to acquire a series of images, which can be played back in a video model, to visualize structural changes during the cardiac cycle.

TOMOGRAPHIC IMAGING IN MEDICINE

Most modern medical imaging technologies endeavor to produce at least a two-dimensional or a three-dimensional representation of their object. The type of radiation employed and what the signals represent differ among the technologies, while the signal processing and image reconstruction of the digitized data are highly similar. X-rays, gamma rays, and ultrasound measure absorbed radiation; magnetic resonance, **single photon emission** computed tomography (SPECT), and **positron** emission tomography (PET) signals measure the emission of signals from within the body. Nevertheless, for all imaging modes, the reconstruction processes use digitized data from detectors containing position-dependent information. Two-dimensional sections at individual depths are produced by a computation called **back projection**, which forms an image that mathematically attempts to recreate the radiation emanating from the subject at that depth. Because the operation assumes perfect reversibility of the process, the resultant image is blurry. To sharpen the image by correcting for events that alter the path of the photon on the way to the detector, the raw image data is processed, or filtered mathematically before back projecting. Various filters, or **kernels**—a mathematical term—are designed to accentuate particular characteristics of the image. Bone and soft tissue kernels are applied to adjust contrast between different tissue densities or resolution for detecting metastases, respectively.

Three-dimensional images are created by computerized stacking of sections in a process called **multiplanar reconstruction**. Resolution in the x-y plane (head to toe, left to right side for a whole-body scan) is governed by the **pixel** size represented by the detectors, while the z-resolution (top to bottom) is limited by how data are collected from different depths in the subject or the thickness of the slice. Slice thickness depends on the radiation modality being imaged as well as the requirements of the physician for a specific type of information.

CHAPTER 7

Imaging the Light from Within—SPECT and PET

In the spring of 1896, shortly after Roentgens's report of the discovery of X-rays, French physicist Antoine-Henri Becquerel was searching for Roentgen's mysterious X-ray "emanations" in the phosphorescence of uranium minerals exposed to sunlight. Frustrated by the cloudy weather, he tossed the rocks into a drawer. When he later developed sealed photographic plates stored in the same dark drawer, he found darkened images of the rocks on the plates. Curious, he continued experimenting to follow up on his discovery of this strange phenomenon, the first evidence of natural radioactivity. The term "radioactivity" was coined in 1898 by Marie and Pierre Curie to describe the invisible emissions from the two elements (polonium and radium) that they purified from pitchblende, the ore from which the uranium had been extracted. Becquerel's discovery did not have the same initial impact as Roentgen's; the images produced by the more penetrating radiation from the radioactive samples were fuzzier. Ultimately, though, the study of radioactivity led to a much deeper understanding of the nature of the atom.

The natural radioactivity of uranium proved useful well beyond its novelty. The processes of radioactive decay provided physicists an experimental window into the subatomic world. George Hevesy, a Hungarian physicist, following radioactive lead uptake into plants, found in 1911 that radioisotopes were chemically identical to the stable **isotopes** of the same element and that they participated in biochemical and physiological reactions indistinguishably. He showed that the incorporated radioactive elements or tracers "turned over" in cells and organisms, and these elements were replaced over time. This work, which established the utility of

radiotracers in biology and chemistry, earned Hevesy the Chemistry Nobel
Prize in 1943.

The advent of "artificial" radioisotopes generated by the bombardment
of nonradioactive elements with high-energy α-particles or neutrons produced radioactive elements more compatible with biological systems than
naturally occurring radioactive heavy metal ions. Radioactive sodium,
phosphorus, and iodine were soon joined by other elements. Nuclear reactors of the wartime Manhattan Project, besides generating the U-235 and
Pu-239 for the first atomic bombs, also produced a variety of short-lived
isotopes of other elements as a by-product of the nuclear reaction chains.
In 1946, the Atomic Energy Commission announced the availability of
radioisotopes for medical research. This was partly a strategy garnering
continued public support by showing a peace-time use of nuclear power to
the public, even while the military nuclear arms race continued cloaked in
deep secrecy. President Eisenhower's "atoms for peace" program in the
1950s continued this form of public relations.

As a result, radioisotopes became available for medical research,
although imaging was initially not considered a primary application. There
were several reasons for this. The first was technical. Sensitive gamma-ray
cameras did not exist, only the recently invented gas-filled **Geiger-Muller
tube**, which relied on the ionization of the gas by high-energy gamma
rays, a relatively inefficient process. It also did not provide precise direc-
tional information about the location of the source. The second was conceptual. Measuring the distribution of radioisotope after it had been
introduced into the body was not an image in the traditional sense in that it
did not represent a picture of an organ, but the functional space into which
the tracer could penetrate and remain during the measurement. People
were not used to thinking in those terms. The tracer nature of radioisotopes
provided a diagnostic modality that was unique. Imaging technologies
allowed physicians to see structural anatomy, whereas introduced radioisotopes could, if the molecules to which they were attached were appropriately designed, provide previously unobtainable functional measures of
physiology in the living organism. Structural and functional images from
multiple imaging modalities now are routinely overlaid to help physicians
integrate the different types of information to aid clinical interpretation.

Hevesy's 1935 studies with rats illustrated selected targeting of
radioisotopes of elements by showing that certain natural radioisotopes
were retained or concentrated in particular organs or tissues. This laid
the groundwork for the therapeutic uses of isotopes, such as iodine that
accumulate in the thyroid gland to target tumors in that organ. The
production of an isotope of technetium (^{99m}Tc) in the cyclotron near

the end of the 1930s provided an isotope with an appropriate energy and convenient radioactive decay **half-life** for biological imaging. This metal ion isotope, a **radionuclide**, was suitable for multiple studies because it was taken up by many different tissues, although this prom-iscuity could lead to difficulties in interpretation. ^{99m}Tc use became routine in 1961 after chemists prepared a sequestered form of the metal ion that they could attach to other molecules that would target the radi-oactive complex specifically to a desired organ or tissue. These radio-pharmaceuticals meant that physicians no longer had to rely on the natural affinity of the radioactive tracer for an organ or tissue, but were limited only by the ingenuity of the radiochemists to synthesize car-riers, often specific drugs, to provide the requisite selectivity. Eric Sea-borg and J. G. Hamilton used the cyclotron at Berkeley to create useable quantities of radioisotopes of sodium, potassium, chlorine, bro-mine, and longer half-life isotopes of iodine useful in biological stud-ies, which did not exist in appreciable quantities in nature.

While a particular radioisotope may be useful as a chemical tracer in biological experiments, the requirements for the properties of a func-tional imaging agent are more restrictive, and those for a viable clinical imaging probe more stringent still. The radioactive decay mode is im-portant. Particulate radiation, such as alpha particles (helium nuclei) and neutrons, is quickly blocked by nearby molecules. Thus, these molecules have a very short range in water and tissue, and so they do not reach an external detector. In addition, because of their mass, they carry a great deal of energy and interact strongly with molecules in their vicinity, depositing the energy that creates chemical radicals and damaging tissue. High-energy electrons (β-) such as those emitted by the decay of ^{32}P can penetrate a few millimeters in tissue but also are absorbed and initiate free-radical chemistry.

X-rays and gamma photons, as we have seen, possess sufficient energy and interact relatively weakly with water and tissue components, escaping the body to interact with an external detector. Gamma-emitting isotopes have dominated the emission-imaging field. To be useful as imaging agents, the characteristic energy of the gamma photons must be compatible with high-efficiency detectors. The rate of photon production also must be high enough for practical data acquisition times. Finally, the half-life of the radioisotope should be long enough for chemistry to be performed and to allow time for shipping, yet short enough to limit the radiation dose to the subject. Thus, out of the 2,230-plus known radioisotopes of the current 117 elements in the Periodic Table, only a handful are potentially useable for medical imaging.

SINGLE PHOTON EMISSION IMAGING—SPECT AND PET

After the availability of biologically useful isotopes came the development of the machines to detect their distribution in a live patient. Two groups of isotopes emerged that produced gamma photons of sufficient energy to escape the body, yet were compatible with detectors, and would not overly expose the subject to radiation damage. One group produced gamma photons directly in the decay process, while the other produced gamma photons as a consequence of the secondary reaction of a positron **antimatter**-matter **annihilation** event. The coincident generation of gamma photons traveling in opposite directions from the annihilation event eventually proved to give the highest resolution images. However, in early studies, gamma photons were detected identically without regard to what process generated them. Isotopes producing gamma photons by either mechanism were used for clinical studies.

At first, physicians moved a Geiger-Muller tube slowly over the patient injected with radioisotope, listening to the crescendo of clicks as they approached the area emitting the highest concentration of gamma rays. The first organ studied by nuclear medicine was the thyroid, whose high uptake of iodine for the biosynthesis of thyroid hormone was studied in 1938 with ^{128}I made by physicist Enrico Fermi using a neutron source he had built. Physicist Benedict Cassen at the University of California—Los Angeles (UCLA) built the "scintiscanner" in 1951, employing a photomultiplier crystal, a device recently developed for X-ray radiology to rapidly capture fluorographic images. The scintiscanner recorded the intensity of gamma-ray emission as the camera was scanned back and forth across

Table 7.1 Gamma-Emitting SPECT and PET Isotopes Used in Medical Imaging

SPECT		PET		
Isotope	Half-life	Isotope	Half-life	Mean range in water (mm)
^{99m}Tc	6.02h	^{11}C	20.4m	1.1
^{111}In	2.83d	^{13}N	9.96m	1.5
^{123}I	13.2h	^{15}O	2.03m	2.5
^{131}I	8.02d	^{18}F	1.83h	0.6
^{201}Tl	3.04d	^{67}Ga	3.26d	2.9
		^{82}Rb	1.25m	5.9
		^{94m}Tc	53m	9.4
		^{124}I	4.16d	0.8, 1.3

the patient. In 1954, then—University of Pennsylvania medical student David Kuhl developed an improved device that encoded the output from the photomultiplier as intensity of light used to expose film or photographic paper, thus producing images in a medium that radiologists were already used to reading.

Kuhl continued to build improved scanners with later versions by adapting this technology to traditional tomographic principles. He back-projected lines of emission data obtained by rotating the patient in front of a camera onto a film cassette that co-rotated with the patient in a technique called single photon emission tomography (SPET). As in early X-ray tomography, this mechanical method blurred the off-line scattered radiation producing crude pictures without the use of computers. By using computer processing to remove the blurring and the artifacts caused by the scattered radiation, and rotating the camera instead of the patient, Kuhl was able to generate useful crude, but true, three-dimensional images of the concentration distribution of a radioisotope within an organ or tissue transforming SPET into SPECT (C for computed). A number of laboratories, including ones at Massachusetts General Hospital in Boston, Washington University in St. Louis, and the University of California—Berkeley, also were involved in the development of SPECT.

In 1958, Hal Anger at the University of California—Berkeley developed an instrument specifically designed to produce images of gamma emission. Instead of scanning a single detector across the subject, he employed a bank of the new highly gamma-photon-sensitive scintillation detectors teamed with a set of lead-collimating channels that restricted the view of the detectors to the area of the subject directly in front of the camera. Gamma photons, like X-rays, cannot be focused by a lens. The **Anger camera** and the multitude of updated commercial versions beginning in the 1960s became the standard gamma-photon-imaging device. In 1968, with collimators angled to focus on photons emanating from a selected depth within the subject and moving the camera like the old-fashioned mechanical X-ray tomographs, the Tomoscanner produced planar sectional images. By the 1970s, improvements in data-processing speed and electronics extended gamma-photon imaging into real-time tomography. Although improved resolution was achieved, the images were not true reconstructions. They retained a great deal of scattered and background blurring, which complicated their analysis. Current Anger cameras are digital and are capable of both single photon counting (used for SPECT) and coincidence photon counting (used for PET).

Before long, computer sampling and reconstruction techniques replaced mechanical tomographic procedures. Three-dimensional imaging actually was implemented in nuclear medicine before it was used for X-ray imaging. Around 1960, data acquisition and computer processing could not handle the high data rates from X-ray detectors, but they were sufficient for the relatively low data rates of gamma-photon counts from patients.

Niels Lassen in Sweden used SPECT to monitor blood flow in the brain as an indicator of brain activity while volunteers performed various tasks with their hand. He also pioneered the use of **color encoding** in the computer-reconstructed images to provide a fourth dimension of radiation intensity representing brain activity. This way of displaying data, known as **heat plots** (blue [cool] through yellow [warm] to red [hot] to represent low- to high-radiation intensity), has spread to the other imaging modalities to convey quantification in a visual display. It can be difficult to remember that the images generated by the SPECT (and PET) emission technologies do not directly represent the physical entities imaged by X-rays or magnetic resonance imaging (MRI). SPECT and PET are functional measures whose output depends on the identity of the radiolabeled molecules employed.

The SPECT machines unveiled in 1968 were the first clinical devices for emission imaging. Their successors remain relatively inexpensive, are the easiest to use clinically, and are the most widely used, although they are not the highest resolution form of emission nuclear imaging. Technology designed to improve the efficiency and spatial resolution of SPECT relied on instrumentation based on the Compton photoelectric effect used by V. Schonfelder in 1973 for balloon-borne gamma-ray astronomy. Similar technology was originally proposed for imaging solar neutrons by K. Pinkau in 1966 and R. S. White in 1968. The first use of a **Compton camera** in nuclear medicine was described by R. W. Todd and J. M. Nightingale in 1974. A gamma-photon Compton scatters from an electron (hence the camera name) in a position-sensitive solid-state detector, which records the event. The photon continues on to interact with a scintillation detector positioned behind the first detector. Mathematical processing of the relative positions of the events recorded from the two detectors, resulting from the interaction of the single gamma photon, allows calculation of the direction of the original incoming photon. This resolution of a Compton camera is improved with higher energy gamma photons, which is the opposite of regular gamma cameras in which the higher energy gamma photons more readily penetrate the shielding between detector elements and thus increase the background signal.

Standard gamma cameras require stringent collimation to restrict detected photons to a small region directly in front of each detector element. Thick lead separators are used to channel gamma photons parallel to their length and absorb all others. This leads to a drastic reduction in gamma-photon intensity reaching the detector element. The Compton camera avoids the use of collimators as it can determine the direction from which the gamma photon came and computationally filter it out or use it appropriately, making much more efficient use of the photons. Increased camera efficiency also translates to reduced radiation dose and lower subject and operator radiation exposure.

The relatively short list of useable SPECT isotopes have sufficiently long radioactive half-lives that they do not have to be generated on-site and can be readily shipped to hospitals outside of major research centers. The most commonly used isotope in SPECT imaging is ^{99m}Tc. It is readily produced on-site in a device that takes advantage of the decay of the parent molybdenum-99 isotope (2.8 day half-life) to the daughter technicium-99m isotope (6.02 hour half-life). The generator can be "milked" for its ^{99m}Tc by infusion of a saline solution, leaving the parent isotope behind. The ^{99m}Tc metal is then chemically attached to whatever molecule is being used to target the tracer.

Drawbacks to SPECT include low resolution and somewhat extended exposure of patients to low levels of radiation for several days as the relatively long-lived (compared with PET nuclide) radioisotopes decay.

Table 7.2 SPECT Labeled Compounds for Clinical Imaging

^{201}Tl chloride, ^{99m}Tc-setamibi, or ^{99m}Tc-tetrafosmin	myocardial perfusion
^{67}Ga citrate	infection or lymphoma detection
^{99m}Tc chloride	brain lymphoma detection
^{111}In-capromab pentetide	prostate cancer detection
^{99m}Tc-MDP (methylene diphosphonate)	metastasis
^{99m}Tc-HMPAQ (hexamethylenepropylene amine oxime)	brain perfusion
^{99m}Tc-labeled red blood cells	liver hemangioma detection
^{99m}Tc-sulfur colloid	liver and spleen assessment
^{99m}Tc sestamibi or ^{99m}Tc tetrafosmin	parathyroid localization
^{99m}Tc-DTPA	renal cortical glomerular clearance
^{99m}Tc-MAG3 (mercaptoacetyltriglycine)	renal tubular function

These specific deficiencies are overcome by another form of gamma-ray emission imaging in which the gamma photons are a product of a different mode of radioactive decay.

POSITRON EMISSION IMAGING—PET

Positrons (β^+), the antiparticle of the electron (β^-), were predicted by Paul Dirac in 1930 and first reported in cosmic ray decays in 1932 by a young physicist at Caltech, Carl D. Anderson, for which he shared a Nobel Prize in 1936. J. Thibaud and F. Joliet first observed positron emission from radioactive nuclei in 1933 and described the annihilation reaction when that form of antimatter encountered an electron, creating two gamma photons. For imaging purposes, the emission of the two annihilation gamma photons in opposite directions (180 degrees) provided significant advantages in resolution and sensitivity over the single gamma-photon emissions of other radioisotopes used in SPET or SPECT imaging. Collimators that restricted the field of view to localize the source of incoming photons and that reduced sensitivity by blocking photons were no longer required. Coincidence of the time of arrival of the two oppositely directed gamma photons at detectors placed on opposite sides of the subject was sufficient to screen out photons from other decay events or from scattered photons.

The technical requirements of reliably detecting coincident events at high count rates in efficient detectors for the high-energy gamma photons (0.511 million electron **volts** [MeV]) delayed the introduction of instrumentation that could take advantage of the superior resolution of the method. Because the positron-emitting isotopes generate gamma photons, they also can be imaged with SPECT equipment although the advantage of coincidence detection is lost. The early work on noncoincidence detection with these isotopes was carried out with the standard Anger scintillation cameras.

The first use of positrons in medicine was made by C. Tobias in 1945 with ^{11}C-carbon monoxide (CO) studying the elimination of CO from the body using the single photon counting mode, the method available at the time. Positron detectors were put to work on clinical problems at a number of U.S. laboratories during the 1950s, including the Brookhaven National Labs in New York, the Donner Laboratory at Berkeley, and research-oriented medical schools in St. Louis, Los Angeles, and Philadelphia. The concentration of research was dictated by the availability of cyclotrons to produce the short-lived PET isotopes. Michael M. Ter-Pogossian's group at Washington University in

St. Louis built a crude imaging device in 1972, a helmet-like contraption spiked with twenty-six detectors, immediately dubbed the "lead chicken," that produced a crude image because the data was processed manually.

No one at that time had made the conceptual connection between transmission and emission tomography to realize that they were mathematically related, and hence data manipulations developed for transmission tomography could be readily adapted for emission tomography. The connection became apparent with the publication in 1973 of Godfrey Hounsfield's X-ray tomographic (CT) reconstructions. Two junior faculty members in Ter-Pogossian's lab, Michael Phelps and Edward Hoffman, cannibalized the "lead chicken" for parts to build an interconnected array of detectors. After overcoming a variety of engineering and computational obstacles, they used coincidence detection and computer algorithms similar to those used for CT to reconstruct an image slice published in 1975. Phelps and Hoffman later teamed up with Kuhl who had been working on SPECT at the University of Pennsylvania.

In 1979, Kuhl and two of his colleagues, Joanna Fowler and Alfred Wolf, attached the PET isotope fluorine-18 to 2-deoxyglucose, which a former student of Kuhl's had used in 1957 to study glucose uptake in the brain. The new compound, fluorodeoxyglucose (**FDG**), quickly became the most often used PET agent, because it could be used to image metabolic activity in the brain and the fluorine-18 isotope had a more convenient half-life (110 minutes) than carbon-11 (20 minutes). More facilities could use the fluorinated PET **ligand** because it could be shipped from the site of manufacture and did not require an on-site cyclotron for isotope generation. Whereas early physiological studies relied on deficits caused by brain lesions, experimental or otherwise, FDG imaging allowed real-time measurement and localization of metabolism changes within the brain. Neuronal activity is accompanied by a high level of glucose uptake that powers the ionic gradients supporting the nerve impulse.

Subsequent development of radiopharmaceuticals concentrated on developing labeled molecules that would bind to receptors, for example, proteins such as those that controlled **specific ion** channels by binding **neurotransmitters** or other ligands. This allowed researchers and physicians to assess alterations in the amount or distribution of specific receptors in the brain or elsewhere by imaging. Some examples include D2-subtype dopamine ligands used in movement disorders such as Parkinson's disease, opiates for pain but more often for epilepsy, the hormone estradiol for estrogen-dependent tumors, epidermal growth factor for epidermal growth factor-dependent tumors, α_2-adrenergic ligands in hypertension and a variety of neurologic diseases, and peripheral benzo-diazepine receptor ligands for glial cell activation in the brain and neuroin-flammation. A broader spectrum of ligands has been applied in animal models for both basic research and for the development of those ligands for eventual clinical use. SPECT- and PET-labeled ligands and substrates are used to monitor cell proliferation, cell death, and blood flow, as well as cellular chemistry, including activity of enzymes, protein synthesis, and gene expression, all in the living animal. Table 7-2 lists some examples.

CHAPTER 8

Lighting up the Body's Own Molecules—Magnetic Resonance Imaging

Magnetic resonance imaging (MRI) is one of the most useful methods for imaging soft tissue such as the brain, muscle, and internal organs. MRI's high resolution is also useful for detailed analysis of bone, ligaments, and tendons. Studies can be performed on the anatomical scale down to microscopic dimensions (micrometers) in an application called magnetic resonance microscopy, although the imaging time and magnetic field strength required for this level of resolution restricts its utility at this time to animal studies.

Nuclear magnetic resonance spectroscopy (MRS), which was the original form of magnetic resonance, with its roots in the chemical structure of molecules, is not an imaging mode. It was limited to studying molecular structure of purified chemicals dissolved in a solvent in a small glass tube placed in a large magnetic field. Improvements in magnet technology and data analysis have expanded the sensitivity and capability of MRS to the analysis of complex mixtures of molecules. **Metabonomics** is a recent application of MRS to extracts of biofluids and tissue samples in which a fingerprint of signals is related to a physiological or pathological condition. MRS is also used to determine concentrations of specific cellular molecules in live tissue and organs such as muscle and brain, although at present this is currently primarily a research tool.

Magnetic resonance was not originally envisioned as an imaging modality. It required the foresight and unswerving determination of several individuals to make the necessary changes in the way they thought about magnetic resonance. They also possessed the engineering skills to adapt the existing technology to measure and locate differences in the distribution of the magnetic properties of the nuclear matter in a position-sensitive fashion throughout the volume of a sample that could be as large as the human torso.

The Austrian physicist Wolfgang Pauli predicted in 1924 from his mathematical models that the recently discovered protons and neutrons making up atomic nuclei would possess certain magnetic properties. Magnetic resonance technology developed from physics experiments designed to confirm and study those predictions. The magnetic properties of nuclei were first detected in solid hydrogen by two Soviet scientists. Later, U.S. physicist Isidor I. Rabi measured the strength of the magnetic moment, also called "spin" of the proton, for which he received a Nobel Prize in 1944. Observation of the magnetic resonance phenomenon itself was another example of an idea whose time had come. In 1946, Edward Purcell and Felix Bloch reported nearly simultaneously the measurement of a radiofrequency resonance of the hydrogen nuclei of water placed in a strong magnetic field, for which they were jointly awarded a Nobel Prize in 1952.

The resonance frequencies of hydrogen nuclei differed from one another slightly, by a few parts per million, depending on the atom to which they were attached and the chemical structure of the molecule of which that atom was a part. The first uses of nuclear magnetic resonance (NMR) were in physics and chemistry. The exquisite sensitivity to the chemical structure of the molecule and to the proximity of other nuclear spins made it a standard method in the armamentarium for structure determination of molecules. The nuclear resonances of individual protons in a molecule could be separated on a frequency scale producing a characteristic fingerprint called a spectrum. Isotopes of elements other than hydrogen were also found to have nuclear magnetic properties, further expanding the utility of the resonance method.

Into the 1950s, the main use of NMR was in studying the chemical structures of molecules. NMR spectroscopy was a tremendous boon to synthetic chemists who could now rapidly determine molecular structures of the new compounds that they made, even in mixtures, without laboriously crystallizing the individual compounds and performing X-ray diffraction. Before computers, X-ray crystallography required pages of mind-numbing calculations, and not all compounds yielded useful crystals. NMR can be performed on solids, a favorite state of matter for physicists. The structural organization of molecules within a solid can be determined on a microscopic scale, although this uses principles more akin to those of the spectroscopy used in chemistry than those involved in MRI.

How was a method that was so well suited for determining the structure of single molecules harnessed to visualize anatomical structures in the human body? The storyline of the development of MRI required the confluence of technological development and the desire on the part, mainly, of two individuals to apply a tool for physicists and chemists to biological systems. Through their pioneering efforts, NMR methods were transformed from purely analytical molecular tools of interest primarily to physicists and chemists into a powerful biological imaging and functional technology. This method filled a gap in the medical need to obtain high-resolution information about soft tissues that were relatively transparent to X-rays.

Much as in the development of ultrasound imaging, two dichotomous biological uses were first envisioned for the technology. Raymond Damadian, a research physician at New York's Downstate Medical School in Brooklyn, tested the theory of Gilbert Ling that the water structure in cancer tumors was different from that in normal cells. Because NMR was highly sensitive to the structure of molecules and water was the molecule in highest concentration in soft biological tissues, Damadian wanted to measure NMR parameters called T1 and T2 on pieces of freshly excised cancerous and normal tissue from rats. Lacking proper instrumentation in his own laboratory, he took his experiment to a small company called NMR Specialties, a spinoff from the main Varian Company, producer of NMR machines for chemical studies, and found in 1970 that the water signal of cancerous tissue was distinctly different from normal tissue.

After publishing his results the following year, Damadian set about to build an NMR machine large enough to contain a human. Like physicist William Fry and his wife Elizabeth Kelly-Fry in Illinois and the Englishman John Wild in Minnesota with the ultrasound method, Damadian envisioned biological NMR primarily as a diagnostic device to detect cancerous cells and filed for a patent on the concept in 1972. He wanted to detect cancers and was less interested, as least initially, in obtaining fine anatomical detail. Although he constantly swam against prevailing scientific opinion and battled a lack of funding, Damadian and his band of committed followers bolted past the usual painstaking incremental progression of scale-up testing through animal models and concerns about the safety of powerful magnetic fields to build a machine that could hold a human.

While others in the magnetic resonance community were using permanent or iron-core electromagnets magnets to generate their magnetic fields, Damadian employed a fledgling magnetic technology to generate an extremely strong magnet that bypassed the field strength limit of the earlier systems. He creating an electromagnet whose field-generating coils were cooled with liquid helium to a temperature near absolute zero. At this temperature, their electrical resistance disappeared and they became superconductors. This produced magnetic field strengths and thus sensitivities many times higher than his competitors. He called his body-sized NMR machine *Indomitable* (Kleinfield 1985) and revealed it to the public in 1977. *Indomitable* was designed to determine whether a tumor was present in the sample volume, that is, the part of the body in the active part of the magnet within the wire coils that detected the radiofrequency resonance. As originally conceived, this was not an imaging instrument. It did not provide any spatial information about the anatomical location of the tumor.

The man who is credited with bringing imaging together with magnetic resonance was engineer and chemist, Paul Lauterbur. The Ohio native first learned about NMR in 1951 while he was pursuing his graduate degree from the Mellon Institute in Pittsburgh and working for Dow Chemical Company, and then again during his service in the military labs in Maryland. After his military obligation, he joined the faculty at State University New York−Stoneybrook in 1963 and then moved to head NMR Specialties in 1971, the same company that allowed Damadian to use their NMR instrument for his tumor measurements. Looking at Damadian's results in the summer of 1971, Lauterbur felt that there had to be a better way to get the information than cutting off samples of tissues to put in an NMR machine.

That solution came to him one night when he realized that the distorted NMR spectrum of a chemical sample in a poorly tuned magnet, one with an inhomogeneous field, carried information both about the sample and the magnetic field. Chemists normally make the field as homogeneous as possible and even spin the sample to average out any remaining inhomogeneities. What if he could make the magnetic field vary in a predictable way across the sample? Because the resonance frequency of the sample is proportional to the magnetic field strength, Lauterbur could determine where in the sample the resonance occurred. If he then changed the direction of the magnetic field gradient slightly and ran the resonance experiment again, and repeated this many times, he could build up an image of the spatial distribution of the resonance in the sample.

After a few days, he had figured out the mathematical manipulations required to reconstruct an image from the resonance signals, which turned out to be similar to Hounsfield's later method for CT. He called his new technique **zeugmatography**, from the Greek *zeugma*—"to join together"—referring to the magnetic field gradient and radiofrequency resonance. After a frustrating attempt with the university to file a patent on the technology (it was considered not commercially viable and would not recover the cost of filing the patent), it took until 1973 before his paper was published. This was a year before the first CT X-ray machine was marketed by EMI.

Lauterbur's article attracted a great deal of attention from both physicists and the medical community. What remained was to reduce the ideas and crude devices to routine practice. Not only were there significant technical issues to be solved, but CT imaging was already established as a gold standard, and it was producing ever-improving images. The physicist Peter Mansfield at the University of Nottingham in England was unaware of Lauterbur's findings when he began developing methods to image solids at what he hoped would eventually be the atomic level. He independently came up with the magnetic field gradient method to provide spatial definition, but most important, he devised a mathematical representation for the data called a k-space matrix that efficiently stored data and could be rapidly processed to extract three-dimensional positional information. This form of processing was particularly suited for the data produced by the NMR experiment, supplanting the back projection approach used for CT. Mansfield focused on speed in image acquisition, even attempting to develop methods to directly acquire data in all three dimensions simultaneously, bypassing time-consuming reconstruction from individual slices. Lauterbur and Mansfield shared the 2003 Nobel Prize for Physiology or Medicine for the development of the principles of MRI. Raymond Damadian was conspicuously omitted from the award.

The prior success of CT scanning proved critical for the development of MRI. Physicians were eager to apply this new technology for soft tissue analysis to image conditions that were ill-defined or invisible to X-rays. Near the end of the 1970s, NMR lost the nuclear moniker, a casualty of the Cold War and the atomic weapons arms race, to avoid possible patient confusion with radioactivity, and became known as MRI.

The U.S. federal government declined to invest in the development of new MRI instrumentation, leaving the task to private companies such as Siemens and General Electric who had also been involved in the development of CT scanners. Damadian in 1974, after Lauterbur's publication, was awarded patents on cancer detection and an imaging protocol. In 1977, the same year that he unveiled his whole-body NMR device, *Indomitable*, he started a company, FONAR, to commercialize the technology, in part because of the difficulty in obtaining government grants to do so. By 1981, the group led by Alex Margulis, the chairman of the Department of Radiology at the medical school of the University of California–San Francisco, and physicist Leon Kaufman reached the threshold with MRI resolution and sensitivity for clinical applications. They had developed an instrument that achieved millimeter resolution whole-body MRI images with funding from a variety of nongovernmental sources, including the Pfizer Corporation. Thus, by the early 1980s, most of the basic instrumentation and the theoretical foundations of MRI had been developed. MRI, however, continued to be designated an experimental procedure as defined by the Food and Drug Administration (FDA) until 1985, which prevented reimbursement by Medicare and most private insurers. After finally receiving the blessing of the FDA, companies jockeyed for position in clinical MRI instrument development. FONAR was embroiled in a continuous series of patent infringement suits against other MRI instrument manufacturers until October 1997, when it eventually won a judgment against General Electric.

fMRI—Fast MRI or Functional MRI?

Anatomical tomographic MRI, like CT, is susceptible to motion artifacts that distort the acquired image. This difficulty is far more acute with MRI because the time required to accumulate enough signal for an image is considerably longer than for X-rays. Seriously ill or claustrophobic patients and children often find it difficult to remain still within the cramped confines of the magnet long enough to complete the data collection. To deal with the claustrophobia, other magnet configurations such as an open magnet have been commercialized, although they are not useable for all MRI procedures. The programmed changes in the field gradients applied to define the image and the radiofrequency pulse sequences used to excite and detect the magnetic resonance signals generate a considerable amount of noise, which also can be disturbing to some patients.

A portion of the imaging time required can be reduced by improvements in instrumentation—faster computers and computational algorithms speeding data acquisition, or higher magnetic fields that increase the signal intensity, although nature places certain fundamental physical limits on making the measurements. Gains in shortening acquisition time were accomplished by improvements on Peter Mansfield's 1977 echo-planar method of collecting data. In this method, data are collected at multiple points throughout a whole plane through the subject at once, rather than as a single line of data, which gave one point (pixel) in the image. The enhancement in speed provided the ability to generate a series of static images that revealed changes in the distribution of the water signal on the time scale of physiological processes such as blood flow, heartbeat, and intestinal motion, much like the shadowy X-ray pictures flickering across fluoroscopy screens, or kinetic mode CT imaging. Although resolution was reduced by some of the compromises required for speed, fast MRI (fMRI) technology turned out to be useful well beyond simply decreasing imaging time and removing motion artifacts.

fMRI can also stand for functional MRI, in which biological function is overlaid on an anatomical image. Seiji Ogawa, a physicist at Bell Labs in New Jersey, demonstrated in 1989 that the oxygenation state of hemoglobin in the blood in the brains of rats affected the NMR signal from water molecules in the vicinity of that deoxygenated hemoglobin. The removal of the oxygen bound to the iron atom in (oxy)hemoglobin as a result of metabolic activity made the deoxyhemoglobin molecule **paramagnetic**. This made the deoxyhemoglobin molecule act like a small magnet, increasing the proton signal intensity from nearby water molecules tremendously. Ogawa called this phenomenon blood oxygenation level-dependence (BOLD). In collaboration with investigators at the University of Minnesota in 1991, he showed that he could discern areas of increased metabolic activity by their uptake of oxygen (increased deoxyhemoglobin content) in the appropriate brains of human volunteers within seconds of when they performed certain tasks or were exposed to visual stimuli. While other methods of enhancing MRI information content, such as injecting an artificial "contrast agent" such as paramagnetic complexes of ions like gadolinium, are used to enhance differences between tissue elements, the endogenous BOLD method does not require the introduction of any agent.

The BOLD phenomenon was actually causing one of the artifacts that early MRI had to eliminate to accurately display anatomy. Blood flow into and out of organs caused distortion of signals. With the understanding of the mechanism behind the spurious signals, investigators have developed sophisticated specialized methods to use BOLD signals to image and quantify blood flow in the vasculature overlaid onto the structure of the surrounding anatomy.

MRI Contrast Agents

The sensitivity of nuclear magnetic moments to magnetic fields in their vicinity provides opportunity for signal modulation by administering agents that perturb the physical mechanisms of signal generation. Rather than interfering with absorption of the exciting radiofrequency irradiation, which is how contrast agents in X-ray or ultrasound produce their effects, the magnetic moments of the artificial MRI contrast reagents change the characteristics of the nuclear resonance to affect the water signal in the immediate vicinity of the contrast reagent and thus influence the image. Subtraction of images recorded in the presence and absence of contrast agent highlights the changes caused by the agent, often in blood vessels.

Electron Paramagnetic Resonance

The electron also possesses a magnetic moment, even larger than that of the proton, but it can be observed only when it is not paired with another electron in the same orbital. Electrons in stable atoms and chemical bonds shared between atoms in molecules are paired in orbitals such that their magnetic moments cancel. Only when an electron exists unpaired in a radical ion or in the orbital structure of some metal ions, such as copper, cobalt, manganese, nickel, or iron, is **electron paramagnetic resonance** (EPR) observed. Because of the toxicity of an excess of these metals, the body has mechanisms for controlling their exposure to cells. Radicals produced in normal body constituents by leakage from energy production, pathologic processes such as oxidative stress, or exposure to ionizing radiation are also sequestered with varying levels of efficiency. Because of their disturbed electronic structure, most of these radicals are usually highly chemically reactive. They do not survive long before they combine with other molecules, causing damage, including chain reactions forming more radicals, which can be toxic to biological systems.

Physicians and scientists have been interested in following free radical production because of changes that occur due to aging and in some disease states. Because of the greater magnitude of the free electron magnetic moment (1,837 times greater than the proton), the signals will be proportionally greater at a given magnetic field strength, and thus the technique will be more sensitive than NMR. Low sensitivity governed by the physics of magnetic resonance is a major reason that medical imaging is primarily limited to the most abundant molecule, water. The low abundance of free radicals, coupled with technical difficulties because the observation frequency for free electrons is proportionally increased from the radio frequency (MHz) into the microwave region (GHz), has hindered applications in clinical imaging. Localization of EPR signals has been demonstrated in experimental systems, but it has not been developed into a medical imaging modality.

CHAPTER 9

From Oceans and Bathtubs—Diagnostic Ultrasound Imaging

Of all of the modes of imaging adopted for medical purposes, ultrasound holds the longevity record. Seeing with sound has been around for millions of years. Whales, porpoises, moles, bats, and some grasshoppers have been confidently squeaking and pinging their way around in low-visibility environments. They locate obstacles and potential food items with great speed and precision. A bat can locate, pursue, and capture a flying insect in complete darkness guided by bursts of high frequency, 100 kHz (100,000 Hz) sound, far above 20 kHz, the highest frequency of human hearing and above that of the dog whistle. Humans have only recently learned how to create and detect high-frequency sounds and employ them in useful ways.

The first device capable of generating ultrasound in a controlled manner was produced by Pierre Langevin, a former student of Pierre Curie. Pierre and his older brother Jacques had first described the physics of certain kinds of crystals that changed shape in an electric field in 1877. Langevin stimulated a quartz crystal at high frequency with an oscillating electrical field driven by an alternating electrical current. The rapidly expanding and contracting crystal created a series of waves matching the frequency of the oscillating electric field in whatever medium the vibrating crystal was immersed (e.g., air or water).

In contrast to X-rays, which are an electromagnetic wave that does not require a physical medium to propagate, a physical wave in a displaceable material is a sound wave. Langevin found that sound in general, and particularly frequencies above the range of human hearing, or ultrasound, was transmitted easily through water. He tried in 1917 to develop a way to use ultrasound to detect the German submarines that were wreaking havoc on Allied shipping during World War I. The war ended before he had a workable field design. Ultrasound technology, pioneered by S. Y. Sokolov in the Soviet Union, was then used to detect manufacturing flaws in metal objects. An engineer at the University of Michigan, Floyd Firestone, invented the Reflectascope, which worked in water and combined the sound transmitter and receiver in the same device. This advance paved the way for the development of equipment that could be deployed in the field. A variety of difficulties were worked out between the two world wars and sound navigation and ranging (SONAR) was an important contributor to anti-submarine defenses during World War II.

Medical imaging with ultrasound was first attempted in 1937 by the Dussik brothers, Friedreich, a physicist, and Karl, a neurologist, who tried to image the fluid-filled ventricles in the brain of a patient. They measured the transmitted sound, much like physicians transmitted X-rays to form an image on film or fluorescent screen. As was the case for transmission X-rays, the bone of the skull doomed this experiment as did the technical problems of the steep attenuation of the sound signal as it passed through brain tissue. The outbreak of World War II interrupted the medical work but greatly accelerated development of ultrasound technology, bringing to the fore pulse-echo reflection methods for detection of distant objects in water. Detecting the ultrasound reflected from different tissue interfaces rather than measuring the amount transmitted through the tissue turned out to be the key to obtaining useful images, although significant difficulties remained to be overcome.

After the war, several groups developed new pulse-echo techniques to image the human brain, but they were stymied by distortions caused by the bony skull and gave up. Other groups applying the technology to different domains were more successful. Two groups in the late 1940s and 1950s focused on using ultrasound to remedy the diagnostic blind spot of the insensitivity of X-rays to abnormalities in soft tissue. The American physicist William Fry and his wife Elizabeth Kelly-Fry in Illinois and the Englishman John Wild, a physician in Minnesota, concentrated on detecting cancerous lesions, which they found gave a distinctive return-echo signature. Wild favored the pulse technology because he was wary of injuring patients with sustained blasts of ultrasound. Pulsing also allowed him to use the same transducer to send and receive, a configuration that became standard for ultrasound imaging. In the mid-1950s, he built the first handheld rapidly pulsed transducer that produced live images for surgeons readying a patient for cancer surgery.

Douglas Howry at the University of Colorado Medical Center, a physician who had interned in radiology, took a different approach. Trained and practicing as a radiologist, he was acutely aware of the deficiencies of X-rays in soft tissue. Instead of cancer detection, Howry pursued the mapping of soft tissues to improve the quality of ultrasound anatomical images. He started in 1949 with an instrument he built from war-surplus SONAR equipment and obtained an image of his own thigh. Although the engineering technologies for cancer detection and imaging were similar, their instrumentation emphasized fundamentally different imaging information. Howry and Wild competed for many years. Computer processing of ultrasound signals beginning in the 1970s revolutionized the quality of ultrasound images and introduced three-dimensional display.

The real-time nature of high-repetition rate-pulsed ultrasound imaging was applied to the human heart in 1953 by Helmuth Hertz and Ingle Edler in Sweden. By focusing the data analysis on the part of the image that moved, termed M-mode, structures of the heart could be resolved through the cardiac cycle. Ultrasound imaging was also applied to other dynamic functional features. Shigeo Satomura and Yasuharu Nimura in Japan led the way in determining the speed and direction of blood flow by the changes in the ultrasound frequency (Doppler shift) scattered off of moving red blood cells. Full implementation of **Doppler echocardiography** had to await the mid-1980s advent of false color-flow mapping, which visualized both blood vessel flow velocity and direction. Localized tissue temperature differences and their effect on tissue fluid viscosity, which could indicate early stages of infection, were also accessible to ultrasound imaging.

Although ultrasound is applied to many different conditions, most people encounter ultrasound imaging in the obstetrician's office. In 1961, thousands of birth defects caused by the antinausea drug thalidomide, taken during pregnancy in Great Britain and Germany, spotlighted the need for a way to safely monitor fetal condition. Diagnostic X-rays were used sparingly and only in troubled pregnancies because the effects of ionizing radiation on dividing cells was well appreciated by that time. Ultrasound came into use in obstetrics after 1970 as a safer alternative than X-rays, although through the 1970s it was mostly restricted to problem pregnancies. Few direct studies determined the effect of ultrasound on the human fetus, but by the 1980s, it was routinely used to follow pregnancies, and most insurance programs covered ultrasound exams. Since the 1990s, it has become an institutionalized confirmation of pregnancy. The first baby picture for some 70 percent of American couples is a sonogram. Ironically, legislated mandatory ultrasounds have become an issue in abortions in many states.

Almost all current ultrasound imaging uses repeated pulses of ultrasound to build up an image. This produces depth information by recording the time delay of the sound as it reflects back from interfaces at different depths, much as the granddaddy of ultrasound imaging, SONAR, has been used to measure ocean depths and detect submerged submarines since World War I. Pulse technologies are readily interfaced with modern digital technologies and computer processing, which greatly facilitates data analysis and extraction of information from the returning signal. The time delay between emission of a pulse and receiving the reflected pulse is the time it takes the sound to travel to an interface and back to the receiver. In soft tissue, the down-and-back time is 13 microseconds per centimeter (cm) of depth. Like RADAR and SONAR, the time delay is interpreted as distance (depth) for display. Creating an image with depth and transverse resolution requires modulation of both transmission and reception. Additional information beyond the travel time is carried in the returning signal and can be harvested for specialized purposes.

FLOW ANALYSIS IN DOPPLER ULTRASOUND

An important use of ultrasound is to measure blood flow, and with the use of ultrasound imaging techniques, to localize areas of stagnant or disturbed blood flow. Ultrasound is used to guide vascular surgeons to a blood clot or partly occluded blood vessel. The liquid portion of the blood, the sera, returns a very weak signal by itself. Red blood cells in the blood, typically 7 micrometers (μm) in diameter, are much smaller than the ultrasound wavelength, so they do not reflect sound strongly, but they do interact with the sound wave, shifting the frequency slightly up if they are moving toward the sound source or slightly down if they are moving away from the source. This is in direct analogy to the example of the pitch (frequency) of a train whistle appearing to rise to an observer as the train approaches then decreasing as the train passes by, a phenomenon described by C. J. Doppler in 1842. Astronomers use a similar technique with electromagnetic waves (light, radio) to determine how fast a light source such as a galaxy or star is moving toward or away from Earth. To detect the motion, the transmitted sound wave is electronically mixed with the reflected wave to produce a "beat frequency," which is the difference between the frequencies of the two waves and is proportional to the velocity difference. Restriction of reflected signal collection to a narrow time window after transmission defines the depth of that source. Collection of data from multiple depths followed by signal processing and computer manipulation produces a four-dimensional image, the three usual spatial dimensions, and a false-colored image reporting flow direction and velocity. A variety of methodologies have been applied to this basic theme to enhance particular kinds of information, depending on what the clinician is trying to evaluate.

Although finely detailed images obtained by a variety of technologies provide a way to assess the structural integrity of tissue and organs, deficiencies in function may not be visible. Functions such as the cardiac cycle or bowel activity require specific forms of motion or a particular pattern of repetitive activity. In routine use, most imaging modalities produce static images or snapshots that are degraded by significant amounts of motion. Considerable effort is invested to remove the blur caused by motion. Versions capable of rapid imaging to capture data throughout the motion cycle have been developed; however, some compromises usually are required. **Ultrasonography** is intrinsically a real-time imaging modality with a frequently refreshed image suitable for time-dependent measurements of the position of reflecting surfaces within the subject.

ULTRASOUND CONTRAST AGENTS

Although ultrasound is much better than X-rays at discriminating small difference in soft tissue density, some anatomical structures of interest remain difficult to distinguish. As for the other imaging modalities, physicians have found it useful to introduce agents that increase the difference between an object of interest and the surrounding tissue. An ultrasound contrast agent must have selectivity for the tissue of interest, be stable during the observation period, possess low toxicity, and be eliminated safely from the body.

A liquid-gas interface is highly reflective of ultrasound and can interfere with ultrasound imaging. Gas trapped in the bowel will often obscure tissue detail beneath. Oral administration of a contrast agent with appropriate bulk and cohesiveness such as cellulose is used to displace that gas to allow visualization of intestinal and stomach wall structure and integrity. An ultrasound contrast agent, on the other hand, takes advantage of the reflectivity of gas. Tiny gas bubbles with radii around 3 μm injected into the circulation efficiently scatter typical diagnostic ultrasound frequencies. If the bubbles are larger than 6 μm in radius, they will be removed in the lung capillary bed. Encapsulation of the gas bubble with a thin coating of different materials increases their stability and reduces diffusion of the gas into the liquid phase, which decreases bubble size. The coating can be engineered by incorporating additives to cause the bubble to be retained in particular locations. Applications of these contrast agents include imaging of the chambers of the heart, and vasculature of the heart, liver, breast, and kidney. Tumor vascularity also can be determined, allowing the identification of tumor type.

A variety of techniques are used to derive information from the infusion of an ultrasound contrast agent. A brief higher-power ultrasound pulse directed to a localized area will break down the bubbles in that region, allowing the measurement of reperfusion as a fresh supply of bubbles flow into the area from the circulation. A subtraction image can be formed from the contrast-enhanced image before and immediately after the high-power pulse, thus removing any background signals and leaving only the scattering from the infused contrast reagent. Deep-lying blood vessels containing the bubbles are otherwise obscured but become visible under these conditions.

WHAT IS AN ULTRASOUND IMAGE?

Since the properties being reported by the returning ultrasound waves are different from those reported by visible light, the ultrasound image does not necessarily look like what our eyes would see if the skin were removed. Sonographers learn to interpret the output on the screen or film much as radiographers learn to interpret X-ray films. Interpreting an obstetric sonogram of a fetus is an art and a skill. Few ultrasound technicians or physicians can render an accurate interpretation of the blurry image. Parents-to-be need help in recognizing anything in their first glimpse of their *in utero* developing child in the prenatal ultrasound image. Like with a Rorschach blot, the observer sees what they want to see or are told is visible. Experts can find the fetal brain and heart and locate defects. The detailed and readily recognizable published high-resolution ultrasound images of fetuses (usually high-risk pregnancies) are acquired with special intravaginal transducers and modified image-processing technology.

CHAPTER 10

Shining a Light Within—Endoscopy

As useful as the other medical imaging modalities can be for a physician seeking diagnostic information on a patient, MRI, X-ray, and emission imaging give physicians senses that they have had to learn to interpret. In return they get important structural information, some of it of the inside of organs or tissue masses, and functional parameters. However, for some situations, nothing is as intuitive or satisfies as well as a visible light image. Surgeons planning an operation want to see with their own eyes what they are dealing with. Since the advent of medical imaging technologies, the days of exploratory surgery to plan an operation are, for the vast majority of cases, a thing of the past. The development of "scoping" surgical technology that allowed physicians to see inside body cavities without general surgery presented the opportunity for surgeons to develop techniques combining observation with the ability to obtain diagnostic samples or remove or repair damaged tissue with minimal trauma to the patient. Laparoscopy (abdomen, pelvic cavity), thoracoscopy (chest cavity), and arthroscopy (joints, knee, elbow) are all forms of **endoscopy** generally performed through a 0.5–1 cm incision. The first laparoscopic operation was reported in 1910 by H. C. Jacobaeus of Sweden and used a crude optical system on a rigid probe. Basil Hirschowitz used the first endoscope with flexible optical fibers to transmit light in and the image out in 1961. Subsequent incorporation of a video camera into the system freed the surgeon's hands.

Endoscopic surgery has expanded in scope with miniaturization of equipment and ingenuity in developing surgical protocols extending the reach of the procedures to tissues and organs not previously accessible. Endoscopy for diagnostic purposes, unhampered by the size limitations of surgical instruments has moved far beyond the rigid endoscopes or even the relatively flexible optical fiber endoscopes. Pill-size video cameras that are swallowed are connected by millimeter-diameter fibers to collect high-resolution pictures of the upper digestive tract.

A wireless endoscopic camera the size of a large vitamin pill that can be swallowed was developed in 2001 by Gavriel Iddan of Given Imaging in Israel for imaging inside the gastrointestinal tract, including the previously inaccessible small intestine. While either end of the gastrointestinal tract can be accessed by traditional upper endoscopy or colonoscopy, the middle 20 feet of the small intestine is too convoluted to risk puncturing the intestinal wall. The miniature video camera and light source of the wireless device pass through the tract over a period of eight hours, taking pictures and transmitting the data to an external recorder worn by the patient while they go about their daily activities. This device has documented a higher incidence of Crohn's disease in children. The observations caused physicians to change many diagnoses from ulcerative or indeterminate colitis to Crohn's disease, which altered their clinical management and improved patient outcomes. Another version with two cameras in the same device is designed to image the esophagus to look for lesions such as those caused by esophageal reflux of stomach acid.

Significantly reducing the size of imaging devices required changing the paradigm and moving away from the standard notion of a camera. Harnessing the physics of optical image generation, Devir Yelin and co-investigators used multispectral interferometry to produce video-rate high-resolution images (Yelin et al. 2006, 2007).

The required components of a device capable of generating high-speed three-dimensional images were incorporated into a probe the thickness ($\sim$350 μm) of a human hair. The data are transmitted back through an optical fiber for computer analysis outside of the body. Although this technology is still in the demonstrative phase, the investigators imaged metastatic tumor nodules on the ovary of a living mouse, introducing the probe into the abdomen through a small needle-size (twenty-three-gauge) cannula. The multispectral nature of the data lends itself to potential future development in analyzing specific spectral characteristics of the imaged region, including exogenously added agents that probe the presence and distribution of specific molecules, such as a tumor antigen, analogous to the specific radioligands imaged in PET and SPECT emission imaging.

Besides providing real-time observation for physicians, computer-based image reconstruction techniques similar to those applied in other areas of medical imaging are used to generate three-dimensional images. In addition, the human brain is able to extract image perspective from the multiple views provided by the video streaming of images, which are lacking in single frames. Processing of the video data using techniques common to the other medical imaging modalities can produce similar three-dimensional renderings, which can be viewed from multiple angles.

CHAPTER 11

Future Imaging Modalities

Present medical imaging modalities range across the gamut of electromagnetic and physical energies that are compatible with our water-filled and somewhat-delicate bodies. A primary limitation for imaging is sufficient resolution to localize or map the property of interest in a useful way onto the dimensions of body components. Future imaging modalities are likely to be measures of function rather than of anatomy. Being able to make functional measurements, particularly if they can be localized in space inside the intact human body, reduces the amount of diagnostic guessing that a physician has to make, in which cases he or she infers the functioning of internal organs from external signs with the aid of a few lab values.

Many functional properties in the living body are connected to ion flows that generate local electrical and magnetic fields. Dead or dying tissue lacks or has reduced ion flow. The fields can be picked up by properly placed highly sensitive external sensors. Most readily detected are groups of units that normally function synchronously producing an integrated signal that varies with time, such as an **electroencephalogram** (EEG, brain waves from groups of neurons) or **electrocardiogram** (EKG, heart muscle electrical activity). The two-dimensional (signal versus time) strip chart recording or computerized equivalent of these field changes is a temporal rather than a spatial image that is the product of multiple detectors. These technologies are thus outside the scope of medical imaging as it is currently practiced. Because there is utility in being able to physically localize alterations in the average signals being recorded, technologists are investing considerable effort in finding ways of producing medically useful images from those signals. For example, a neurosurgeon would be greatly assisted by an image that localized exactly where in the brain of a patient an epileptogenic focus wreaked its excitatory damage. Standing in the way of converting this information into a three-dimensional image are a number of technical challenges as well as the need to develop ways of deriving the kind of information needed for image reconstruction. The process is not as straightforward as that used for the standard imaging modalities, because the ray-tracing methods common to their analysis do not apply to the integrated electrical signals. The most developed example of the promise and the problems of these new modalities is provided by measurements of impedance that reflect the electric fields produced by ion flows.

THE STATE OF IMPEDANCE IMAGING

Bioimpedance refers to the interaction of externally applied electrical currents and their accompanying magnetic fields with an organism. Although the principles are similar, bioimpedance is distinguished from **bioelectricity,** which is electrical currents (and their accompanying magnetic fields) generated within a living organism by the chemical and biochemical processes of life. Bioelectricity is an unavoidable consequence of muscle and nerve activity and the presence of electrochemical gradients of ions and charged metabolites across cellular membranes. Upon death of the organism or the cell, bioelectrical activity ceases as energy sources dissipate and the ionic gradients collapse. Pathological processes can reduce cellular or tissue function, causing abnormalities in the bioelectric signals or in tissue responses to applied fields. Evaluation of these abnormalities, especially the changes in those properties, provides a functional readout of the physiological state of that organ or tissue.

The most familiar bioelectric measurements used in clinical diagnostics are the relatively strong signals from action potentials, the EKG measuring heart function and the EEG measuring brain function. These methods currently are not employed in an imaging mode. The outputs from a series of electrodes are displayed as a series of signal versus time graphs, squiggly lines on real or virtual chart paper. Over the years, characteristic features of these graphs have been collected by physicians and correlated with specific conditions. Specialists are trained to recognize these features, which they use for diagnosis. This is medically effective even though often the physiological basis for the observation is not known.

HISTORY OF BIOIMPEDANCE MEASUREMENT

The interaction of electricity with biological tissue was described several years after Benjamin Franklin's kite experiment of June 1752. Franklin is often given credit for the first demonstration of the phenomenon of electricity. Although lightning was not new, the detail of his observations and the logical framework he constructed to produce a rational explanation were the cornerstone on which others would build a true understanding. Several of the terms he used in his description, such as conduction, charge, and discharge are still used in the twenty-first century. A few years later Luigi Galvani in Bologna, Italy, described "animal electricity" when he made a dead frog's leg jump by applying an electrical current to the nerve. This crude demonstration of electrophysiology became popular in the 1800s in the form of "medical electricity" applied by physicians and quacks alike to patients for a wide variety of real and imagined ailments. Hermann Mullers described the electrical properties of biological tissues, in particular the directionality of current flow in certain tissues, such as muscle. He noticed changes in the reaction to electrical current after excitation and when tissue was damaged by a lack of oxygen.

Developments in membrane biophysics during the 1930s laid the groundwork for understanding the physics of the electrical observations that were being made and for elucidating the contributions of biological molecules in the blood and body fluids. Improvements in technology around the time of World War II by Cole and Fricke made measurements of tiny electrical currents feasible in a clinical setting. Tissue bioimpedance is highly sensitive to volume changes reflecting alterations in water content. J. Nyboer introduced thoracic electrical bioimpedance in 1950 as a noninvasive way to measure cardiac function using a set of four aluminum foil electrodes placed on the arm. In the mid-1960s, W. Kubicek applied arm and thoracic electrodes to NASA's astronauts to monitor cardiac stroke volume and cardiac output during space flight.

There are a variety of diagnostic and therapeutic uses of the measurement and application of bioimpedance and bioelectricity in biology and medicine. Much of this is in the diagnostic arena and is related to function rather than structure. Obtaining sufficiently reproducible measurements free of various electrical and other disturbances has thus far hampered the localization of signals or signal anomalies of medical interest.

Probably the diagnostic application of impedance measurements that most people have come in contact with, although they may not realize it, is in the determination of body composition—the percentage of body fat. At selected frequencies, electrical impedance measurements provide estimates of the total body water, extracellular-intracellular fluid balance, muscle mass, and fat mass. Initially restricted to doctor's offices, the technology is now widespread. It has been incorporated into some home electronic scales for personal monitoring of fitness regimens, sports medicine, or nutritional assessment. Simply standing on a scale (in bare feet) provides a readout of weight and body fat content that can be personalized to show the optimum for the subject's gender, age, and height.

Other clinically relevant applications utilize bioelectrical impedance. Even without imaging, useful information can be gleaned from tissue electrical signals and responses. EEGs record electrical activity patterns of the 10^{11} neurons in the brain on the order of 50 microvolts (μV) from the skin covering the skull using a network of electrodes. Some spatial localization of the activity is possible with the standard set of twenty-one electrodes so that function or dysfunction of specific brain areas can be determined. The amplitude and frequency of the signals in different functional states induced by sights or sounds or mental activity are characteristic as are the patterns during the different stages of sleep.

Electromyography (EMG) is used to monitor muscle function and nerve-muscle connectivity in certain degenerative muscle conditions. The signals here are much greater, reaching several millivolts (mV) (in contrast to tens of microvolts from the brain) with skin electrodes, because the muscles are close to the surface and the muscle groups relatively large.

Electroneurography of nerve bundles can be monitored with skin electrodes, while single-nerve fibers can be measured with needle electrodes. Stimulation can be performed transcutaneously or via needle electrodes and responses recorded via the EMG electrodes. The measured responses are important in nerve conduction velocity studies in demyelinating neuropathies, such as the constellation of Charcot-Marie-Tooth diseases.

Electrical stimulation is also used as a therapeutic modality. Familiar uses are cardiac pacing (pacemakers) and defibrillation. Also common is transcutaneous electric nerve stimulation (TENS) for pain relief in which the electrical impulse is applied through skin surface electrodes. Because the output from pain sensory nerves requires greater stimulation voltage than the sensory and motor nerves, sensory and motor nerves can be stimulated without activating the pain signaling. Pain relief operates by several mechanisms, including acting on the gating of pain perception in the central nervous system (CNS) of the spine with high frequency pulses (50−200 Hz) and by activating the release of endogenous pain-numbing **endorphins** with low frequency pulses (2−4 Hz). The latter effect probably occurs in higher nerve centers in the brain distant from the stimulus. Endorphin release is also achieved by the rhythmic (2−4 Hz) movement of acupuncture needles, which also stimulate motor nerve fibers.

Attractive features of impedance measurements include the potential for continuous monitoring at high temporal resolution (millisecond), with relatively simple, portable equipment that can be brought to the patient. The patient is not exposed to ionizing radiation, unlike X-ray technologies (CT, fluorography) or radioisotopic imaging (SPECT, PET). Impedance measurements share simplicity of use and safety with ultrasound techniques, and they measure a functional physiological parameter. The downside to impedance imaging is that its spatial resolution cannot compete with other techniques such as MRI for pinpointing the position of a signal. The computational projection techniques that allow three-dimensional image reconstruction for X-ray, MRI, and SPECT/PET imaging are not strictly applicable, because the low-frequency electrical current does not remain in a single plane, which could be reconstructed slice by slice. Complex mathematical algorithms are required to back-calculate a specific conductivity distribution to form an image. Currently, the solutions to the calculations that define the image are somewhat ambiguous and do not give a clear interpretable result. Generating reliable and reproducible results in human patients free of experimental and computational artifact remains a challenge, and thus the potential of the technology currently remains largely unrealized.

Ironically, Mother Nature developed sensitive, high resolution electrical impedance imaging some 500 million years ago. Certain marine and aquatic fish, sharks, rays, and eels have highly developed electroreception capabilities. Some species transmit pulsed weak electrical fields with which they can identify competitors, mates, and even track tiny prey with a high degree of precision (Engelmann et al. 2008). They can even "cloak" their own electrical signature when in danger (Stoddard and Markham 2008). The mechanisms by which they do this are poorly understood. Mormyrid fish emit weak electrical pulses and somehow interpret the resultant field lines along their body to construct an "image" of their dark murky environment at the river bottom (Pusch et al. 2008). The paddlefish, a denizen of the muddy Mississippi River, prized for its roe much like the sturgeon, uses a flattened extended rostrum studded with gel-filled ampullae sensitive to electrical fields to track down and capture its favorite food, millimeter-size *Daphnia*, using the water flea's own bioelectric signature (Wilkens and Hofmann 2007). Since electroreception is not one of the five human senses, it was the middle of the twentieth century before scientists became aware of the phenomenon and developed sufficiently sensitive instrumentation for use in streams, rivers, and the ocean. It is not clear how or whether an "image" as we understand it is mapped in the brains of these organisms (as are the familiar five senses). Somehow, their nervous system is able to generate a real-time, highly localized three-dimensional representation of their electrical environment. One theory proposes that these fish do not register an intensity image, but rather one that reflects phase differences between the field fluctuations generated by field sources moving relative to one another. Further study of the mechanisms involved could help humans refine their impedance technology to produce useable images.

MEASUREMENT OF TISSUE IMPEDANCE

Movement of electrons in a metal wire is an electrical current. Hans Christian Oersted showed in 1820 that wherever there was movement of electrical charge a corresponding magnetic field was connected with that current. In biological systems, the charge movement is overwhelmingly due to the movement of ions in solution such as sodium, potassium, calcium, and chloride rather than electrons. The greatest charge movements occur during the action potentials in excitable tissues such as muscle (skeletal, cardiac, smooth) and in nerves, so signals from these sources tend to dominate the endogenous bioelectric signal from nonneuromuscular cellular ion flows.

A wealth of information about a biological system can be obtained by applying time-varying voltages (oscillating voltages with frequencies from 20 Hz to 1 MHz) and measuring the induced electric fields. Measurements are dependent on the amount of water in the body. Induced current flow at low frequencies is a result of movement of ions in the extracellular compartment because at low frequencies cellular membranes, which are composed of nonconductive oil-like lipid, act like electric capacitors to block the flow of current. At higher frequencies, the current can pass through the membranes and sample the tissue inside and outside of the cells. The frequency effects on currents depend in detail on the particular tissue and its metabolic state. Therein lays the potential of bioimpedance measurements for imaging physiologic function. Potential clinical applications range from imaging ventilation and pulmonary embolism in the lungs, quantifying cardiac output and blood flow, and early detection of breast tumors to measurement of gastric emptying. Although other imaging modalities provide superior resolution, the major attractions for impedance measurements are the real-time, functional readout and lack of exposure to ionizing radiation. Electrical impedance imaging of the brain has been achieved, but anatomical localization was poor. Some utility was seen for continuous impedance monitoring of intractable epilepsy because of the unpredictability of the seizures. Monitoring with the higher resolution but more invasive EEG with implanted electrodes would be difficult. fMRI, the other imaging method capable of localizing the neural activity changes, requires immobilization of the subject in a large claustrophobia-inducing magnet for long periods of time, which is clearly impractical.

Technological improvements in impedance tomography are moving toward replacing the electrodes attached to the subject to apply or receive currents, which are a major source of artifacts. Instead, isolated planar coils connected to low-noise amplifiers (superconducting quantum interference devices [**SQUID**]) interact with the subject via the tiny magnetic fields induced by the flow of current. Similarly, excitation can be applied through a coil at multiple frequencies to obtain the advantages of differential frequency imaging contrast. A version of impedance imaging combined with MRI (Magnetic Resonance Electrical Impedance Tomography) is in the experimental stages, but it promises to deliver high spatial resolution and contrast.

CHAPTER 12

The Digital Age

TELEMEDICINE AND IMAGING

Telemedicine is a rapidly growing form of medical practice that encompasses a variety of diagnostic and treatment modalities that all rely to some extent on some service rendered by an off-site individual or establishment at which data are transmitted by electronic medium of some sort. Criteria defining a service as telemedical are legislated on a state-by-state basis, but usually are standardized to include only those services reimbursable by payers such as Medicare, state agencies, and insurance plans (Mayo and Kepler 2007). For example, a service rendered by telephone or facsimile generally would not be reimbursable in most states. There are many issues surrounding the ethics and security of medical records flowing freely in cyberspace, as well as quality assurance for outsourcing of image analysis and interpretation, which is expedited by the ease and speed of digital transfer. The latter factor is a major point of friction between maximizing company profits by reducing expenses and U.S. professionals seeing their work sent overseas, where images are interpreted by workers who never encounter the patient and whose qualifications may be difficult to establish. While the government may applaud reducing the cost of the ever-increasing number of imaging sessions prescribed by physicians, the issue of qualifications of outsourced technical expertise to maintain the quality of care transcends the economic issues. Appropriate legislation to address this concern has been more difficult to implement than might be expected considering the importance of credentialed professionals for quality care.

Transfer of most medical imaging output is now electronic, taking advantage of computer systems that are compatible with the digital images produced by current imaging equipment. This includes digitization arising from the nature of the data collection or by digitally scanning the analog output of a standard X-ray film. Managing multiple types of data and different imaging modalities, along with all of the rest of the information about the patient in an accurate and secure fashion to maintain patient privacy, is not a simple process. Transmitting imaging data from instruments of different manufacturers in such a way that it is useable by the widest variety of analysis packages is not as simple as posting a JPEG from your digital camera on the Web or attaching it to an e-mail.

In 1983 a joint committee formed by the American College of Radiology and the National Electrical Manufacturers Association set about to establish a standard to provide the necessary tools for diagnostically accurate representation and processing of medical imaging data to provide an all-encompassing data transfer, storage, and display protocol. The standard they came up with became a protocol called Digital Imaging and Communications in Medicine (**DICOM**). The rules and algorithms are implemented in Picture Archiving and Communications Systems (**PACS**), which are the medical systems hardware and software that actually run digital medical imaging. These include data acquisition, archiving images, and display and manipulation systems used by the radiologists to view the images.

Teleimaging is just one part of a growing worldwide movement toward increased delivery of high-tech and high-level medical care to areas outside population centers, some of which are quite isolated. Even inside the United States in which the physical distances and communication barriers are small compared with Africa, South America, and Australia, significant numbers of people are living in areas where the population density and economic factors will not support a complex and capital-intensive medical establishment. In the past, patients would have to travel long distances to tertiary care centers for diagnosis and treatment, or go without. With an increasingly aging population whose expectations and need for health care and advanced diagnostic services are several times greater than those less than forty years old, the need for alternative modes of delivery becomes progressively more acute. Simply building more clinics, training more physicians, and opening more diagnostic centers with the latest equipment is not a viable answer. At the current level of health care, costs are rising at a rate higher than inflation, or the prices of other goods and services. Remote sources of care, that is, telemedicine, have been projected as one solution to this dilemma.

Although many of the technical obstacles to telemedical imaging have been supplanted by cheaper and faster technology and the expanded reach of the Internet, several issues remain to be dealt with for telemedicine to reach its potential for increasing access to quality state-of-the-art medical diagnosis and care. Five areas were identified by the 2001 Telemedicine Report to Congress: (1) lack of reimbursement; (2) legal issues; (3) safety and standards; (4) privacy, security, and confidentiality; and (5) telecommunications infrastructure (United States Office for the Advancement of Telehealth 2001). Reimbursement for telemedicine outside of Medicare is difficult, and it is restricted within Medicare by such provisos as that traditional health care be inaccessible as in an isolated rural setting. Telehealthcare providers in such situations often are registered nurses and licensed practical nurses who are not eligible for reimbursement.

Not all state health plans (only twenty as of the 2001 report) reimburse telemedical claims. There are legal issues surrounding licensure for practicing telemedicine across state lines. Twenty-six states have some form of legal framework governing the practice. Guidelines for clinical protocols and technical standards for interoperability of systems for patient safety remain to be established for telemedicine. Regulatory oversight is shared by the FDA and the Federal Trade Commission (FTC) and state regulatory agencies, but their interaction is not always seamless and without controversy. Privacy and confidentiality issues are governed by the Health Insurance Portability and Accountability Act of 1996 (HIPAA), which specifically mandates a series of national electronic health transaction standards for secure electronic health data management. Any individual state standards more stringent than the federal standards are allowed to take precedence, and thus telehealthcare providers operating across state or international lines are faced with navigating a hodgepodge of regulations. Consumer privacy over the Internet has been judged by the FTC as lacking in protection despite efforts of the industry to self-regulate. A major obstacle to telemedicine in rural areas is the cost of the telecommunications systems needed, which is spread out over a smaller population than in urban areas. The Federal Communications Commission (FCC) is charged with administering a discount program to make up the difference between urban and rural rates.

Telehealthcare has the potential to expand access to medical services for isolated clients, both rural and urban. It could potentially result in cost savings by making more efficient use of expensive infrastructure, although some satellite centers are likely to be required to avoid penalizing those patients living outside of major population centers by limiting their access. This is particularly pertinent for multimillion-dollar MRI or CT imaging technology. The actions of third-party payers, including the government, will likely influence the extent of any cost savings.

PART II

Controversies in Medical Imaging

Compared with gene therapy or the practice of alternative medical treatment, there has been relatively little controversy over medical imaging. While philosophers may discuss the implications of the psychological effects on body image of exposing the body beneath the skin to view, and computed tomography (CT) scans or magnetic resonance imaging (MRI) may influence the way some artists depict the human form, most of this does not register with the general public. They are more interested in learning whether that lump is a tumor, the severity of the broken arm, or whether the knee has cartilage damage. Two issues, however, have received considerable interest: (1) safety of the technologies and (2) their rising cost.

CHAPTER 13

Radiation Safety and Protection

Low-energy radiation such as ultrasound and radiofrequencies used for MRI generally are not considered hazardous at the power levels used in diagnostic imaging. There is some question about how high magnetic fields affect the body. Clinical MRI fields currently range up to 3 **Tesla** in routine use. Higher fields such as 7.1 Tesla magnets have been used experimentally to create greater sensitivity, higher resolution, and decreased scan times. The maximal magnetic field exposure limit currently set by the Food and Drug Administration (FDA) is 4 Tesla for infants younger than one month and 8 Tesla for others. Significant safety concerns exist for people with magnetically active metal implants of any type, or pacemakers or other implanted electronic devices, such as drug delivery systems that would interact with the magnetic and radiofrequency fields used in MRI.

Outside of these areas, the chief safety concerns have, quite reasonably, focused on imaging modes that utilize "ionizing" radiation, such as X-ray and radioactive emissions. As the term ionizing indicates, the radiation is of an energy that can cause chemical changes in components of the body that later can lead to cancer. Because of the delayed effects of X-ray radiation and the lack of understanding of the physics, it took some time before regulations to enforce safety standards were adopted.

An initially unappreciated feature of the magic properties of the newly discovered and aptly named X-rays to visualize what was beneath the skin was their capacity to cause damage. Practitioners and experimenters exposed daily to the mysterious rays were the first to notice reddening of the skin akin to burns on their hands from exposure to the beam from the X-ray tube. The lesions evolved into wounds that would not heal, and the underlying tissue degraded, eventually requiring amputation, sometimes leading to death from infection in this time before antibiotics. A more insidious form of damage would emerge years later as the mutagenic potential of X-rays expressed itself in various cancers. This delayed reaction was a puzzling phenomenon for the medical profession who was used to treating the immediate effects of a thermal burn or a knife wound. Further confusing the issue was the observation that X-ray exposure was effective at killing preexisting tumors and resolving certain skin conditions. How could X-rays be both good and bad?

BASIS FOR RADIATION DAMAGE

Enough studies had been performed by physicists and biologists in the first two decades of the twentieth century to recognize that electromagnetic radiation above a certain energy induced chemical effects on biological molecules. Ionizing energies of electromagnetic radiation start at the level of ultraviolet light, which is responsible for sunburn and skin cancers. Ionizing radiation includes X-rays, gamma rays, and higher-energy radiation, such as cosmic rays. Although not considered in this book because they are of short range in tissue and thus generally are not useful for medical imaging, particulate radiation derived from other radioactive decay modes (α- and β-emissions) are also ionizing. They cause molecular damage including mutations because of their considerable mass, which they usually deposit within a short distance by crashing into molecules.

When radiation of sufficient energy interacts with a molecule, it causes ejection of one or more electrons leaving behind a highly chemically reactive molecule, a free radical, which will combine with nearby molecules. Likewise, the ejected electron will react with other adjacent molecules altering their structure and activity. The most abundant molecule in tissue is water, so radical components produced from water, such as the highly reactive hydroxyl radical, can react directly or go on to produce a cascade of other chemically reactive molecules. When one of these radicals encounters a deoxyribonucleic acid (DNA) molecule, a protein, or a membrane lipid, it will react, altering the function of that molecule. While cellular repair mechanisms can repair radiation damage from the natural background ionizing radiation from the environment as well as this X-ray-induced damage, some modifications slip through the safety net. Damage to DNA has the potential to generate changes in the genetic code of cells. Most of the damage is repaired before it can cause problems, but again some defects slip through, and repairs are not 100 percent faithful. If the change in the genetic code is in a gene encoding for an essential cell function, the cell will die and be replaced. If the affected gene controls cell growth, however, the cell containing the mutated DNA may no longer be under the constraints that restrict that pancreas cell to remain a pancreas cell in the pancreas, and it will begin to divide uncontrollably, forming a tumor.

Development of Radiation Exposure Standards

By 1911, it was clear that X-ray workers and radium workers were presenting with leukemia, a white blood cell cancer, at rates vastly greater than in the general population. A large fraction of American radiologists had childless marriages and those with children experienced almost a twofold increase in certain types of abnormalities. These statistics engaged the interest of labor unions and insurance companies. It was clear that some sort of standards for exposure to radiation needed to be developed to protect both workers and the patients, but setting limits required an understanding of what was happening with radiation exposure over both the short term and throughout life.

Initially, just measuring radiation dosage was a challenge. Arthur Mutscheller proposed a tolerance dose in 1924 based on empirical observation that an operator of X-ray equipment could sustain over prolonged exposure without subsequent injury. In 1925, the first post—World War I meeting of radiologists was held in London to consider this issue among other topics. Physicists could measure ionizing radiation with sensitive ionization chambers, but these were not suitable for measurements outside a highly controlled laboratory. Hans Wilhelm Geiger, who had worked with Ernest Rutherford on the structure of the atom before the war, built a portable device, subsequently called a Geiger-Muller counter, which could measure radiation intensity. By the 1928 meeting of radiologists in Stockholm, physicians suggested a limit based on exposure called an **erythema dose,** an amount of radiation sufficient to cause reddening of Caucasian skin. An international standard was agreed upon of one-one hundredth of an erythema dose per month. Although it was still an arbitrary measure, it was a useful beginning standard for both radiologists and X-ray equipment manufacturers.

During the 1930s, the Committee on Radiation Safety met with the leading X-ray equipment manufacturers (General Electric, Kelly-Koett, Picker, Standard X-Ray Company, and Westinghouse) to further refine the standard. The tolerance dose was redefined to a minimal dose suspected to have a lasting effect. The companies were to a certain extent worried about the health of their workers, but tougher standards on radiation leakage also forced competitors out of the market. The atomic bomb research during World War II provided a big boost to what came to be called health physics. In 1960, the Atomic Energy Commission directed $49 million (1960 dollars), almost 60 percent of its budget, into research in biology for problems of radiation protection.

The ionizing radiation exposure limits today remain to a certain extent arbitrary because it is difficult to determine an absolute "no effect" dose. In addition to an ionizing radiation background resulting from natural radioactivity and cosmic rays penetrating to Earth, questions have emerged about the time at which an effect can be measured following exposure. People living in Denver are exposed to significantly more cosmic rays because there is less protective atmosphere above them and a higher natural radionuclide content of geological formations in the area. Different animal models respond differently to radiation, and different organs and tissues of the animals react differently. Similar differences exist in humans. Some people are better repairers of radiation damage because they have more active repair mechanisms than others.

The trend in exposure standards continues downward, with the exposure allowed to patients being imaged the least of all, typically 5 to 10 percent allowed to personnel operating the equipment. Allowable exposure of children is lower still. With improvements in imaging technology (more efficient sources, better detectors, better algorithms for improving signal to noise), less radiation can be used to achieve the same result.

CHAPTER 14

Whole-Body CT Scanning for Cancer Detection

Whole-body CT scanning is being marketed as a screening procedure for early detection of cancer in the general population. Since their first introduction in the 1990s, for-profit medical imaging facilities have tapped into this lucrative area (Lee and Brennan 2002). In 2002, 32 million whole-body CT scans were performed. Insurance companies do not pay for these scans, which run between $800 and $1,500, because they are still classified as "experimental" because no trials have yet demonstrated that they are effective. The scans are popular with health conscious baby boomers as they enter middle age because they offer apparent reassurance against greatly feared cancers.

X-ray CT can produce high-resolution three-dimensional images of the absorption of X-rays passing through the body. The ability of the technique to reduce the absorptive contributions from overlying structures for each "slice" removes uninformative density from the image, which includes X-rays scattered by the overlying tissue or organs. This effectively expands the range of X-ray intensities that can be distinguished from one another and allows the method to probe soft tissues with a sensitivity that rivals other methods and that extends well beyond standard two-dimensional absorption images such as a standard chest X-ray.

Spectacular structural images are produced showing great detail of the imaged region. Typically, scans focus on the portion of the body suspected by the physician to be responsible for the patient's condition. The increased sensitivity of CT to differences in tissue density is capable of distinguishing and locating solid tumors in areas of the body previously accessible only by exploratory surgery. This comes at the cost of increased exposure to X-rays, which are an ionizing radiation and thus capable of causing DNA damage, mutations, and thus an enhanced likelihood of tumor induction.

DIAGNOSTIC IMAGING

CT scans with and without introduction of X-ray contrast media have proven useful in patients with a diagnosed disease or in individuals at high risk because of family or health history to precisely determine the location and size of a cancer as well as following its rate of growth and spread. It is also useful for directing biopsies and guiding radiation treatment. As an imaging tool, CT is the method of choice for imaging the brain, spine, pelvis, chest, and abdomen. It has been principally helpful with pancreatic, liver, and lung cancers. It may be moderately effective in detecting colon cancer in at-risk individuals as a "virtual colonoscopy," in comparison to traditional endoscopic visualization (Regge et al. 2009). However, CT will not detect blood-borne tumors (lymphomas) and is not useful for detecting all forms of solid tumors. It is of much less value in detecting prostate or ovarian cancers. Thus, a full-body CT scan has limited utility for general screening of all types of cancers.

Screening Imaging

For CT imaging to be accepted for use as a screening tool in a population of otherwise healthy individuals, it must satisfy a much more stringent set of criteria than diagnostic imaging for at-risk individuals. In a subject with a tumor or at high risk for developing tumors (previous tumor, strong family history), the risk of the procedure is considered acceptable because of the severity of the consequences of having a tumor. A similar level of procedural risk is *not* acceptable in the general population of healthy individuals who have only a slight chance of having a tumor. This is especially true if the technique has a high false-positive rate (detects a tumor when there is not a tumor) or a high false-negative rate (failing to detect an existing tumor). False positives will incur additional anxiety and expense because they will require additional invasive and expensive testing. Most of these will turn out to be benign nodules or noncancerous tumors, or scar tissue from prior infections. Sufficiently skilled radiologists and highly trained technicians with high-quality equipment at major health centers are more likely to be able to distinguish suspicious findings from true positives.

Negative results are potentially harmful because they may produce an unwarranted sense of security, which may cause subjects to forgo regular medical checkups, healthier dietary or other lifestyle changes, or to decline more appropriate screening tests (e.g., Pap smear for cervical cancer). Sufficiently extensive clinical trials have not been carried out to prove the effectiveness of whole-body CT screening for cancer. The studies that have been done are not encouraging. Scans of 86 percent of 1,192 consecutive patients scanned in a community clinic produced positive findings, and 37 percent were referred for further testing (Furtado, Aguirre, and Se 2005). Similar findings were published in 2002 by Casola and colleagues. In this study 10 percent of subjects were told of a potential tumor, but only 1 percent actually had a life-threatening condition.

Cost versus Benefit Analysis

In the absence of full-scale clinical trials, hard numbers are hard to come by. Computer modeling assuming standard prevalence of diseases in the general male population was used to compare a one-time whole-body CT scan to routine methods of detection in a hypothetical group of five hundred thousand men looking for colon, pancreatic, lung, liver, and kidney cancers as well as coronary artery disease and abdominal aortic aneurism. A 90 percent false positive rate necessitating additional testing incurred one-third of the additional cost attributed to the CT method. Only 2 percent had actual disease. An additional expense of $2,513 per person for those receiving the single whole-body CT scan (assumed cost $900 in 2001 dollars) provided an additional six days of life expectancy compared with those receiving routine care. Although the CT scan would be patient-paid, the additional expenses for the 90 percent of the patients requiring follow-up testing would be eligible for payment by insurance (Beinfield 2005), hence adding to health care systems costs.

More focused CT screening for cancer, particularly when applied to populations at risk such as smokers, can be effective. Spiral CT scanning for lung cancer nodules in asymptomatic current or ex-smoking subjects produces cost-benefit numbers on the same order as other screening imaging technologies. It is as effective as mammography for breast cancer (diagnosing 0.6 percent versus 0.5 percent) in the over-fifty smoking population for a similar cost of $30,000–$50,000 per year of life saved. There are more than 80 million current and former smokers in the United States (Henschke et al. 1999). Hence, CT scanning can be of value when appropriate subject populations are analyzed rather than general population screening.

Incidental Findings

Precisely because such a large proportion of the body is being imaged during whole-body CT, the likelihood is high of detecting abnormalities unrelated to the original testing. This issue is discussed under ethics of medical imaging when much more limited anatomical regions are being imaged. What are the responsibilities of the imaging team to report abnormalities, and what are the criteria for abnormality?

Radiation Exposure

The most serious issue of whole-body CT scanning involves the additional health hazard of exposure to additional ionizing radiation. CT's high resolution comes with a cost. It requires considerably higher X-ray doses than other X-ray imaging procedures to generate the three-dimensional image. A single whole-body scan requires an exposure roughly equivalent to 100 mammograms (Brenner and Elliston 2004). Tumor incidence increases with increasing cumulative exposure and is higher the younger the subject is when exposed, presumably because there is a longer time for a cancer to be expressed during the lifetime of a younger person. For a single scan, the incremental increase in tumor incidence would be low, estimated at 1 additional tumor in 1,200–2,000 subjects of age forty-five. When applied in a screening mode in the general population, one scan per year for the ensuing thirty years starting at age forty-five, the incidence of a radiation-induced tumor rises to one in fifty subjects. This is clearly unacceptable in a test for the general population when benefit has not been shown. When used for diagnosis in situations in which there is reason to suspect the presence of a tumor, the ability to detect, locate, and measure the growth rate of the tumor, the metric changes and the scan is well worth the risk. In this situation, the subject's life is in danger from the existing tumor, and the scans can be targeted and significantly fewer are required.

The FDA Web site posts the following statement:

> At this time the FDA knows of no data demonstrating that whole-body CT screening is effective in detecting any particular disease early enough for the disease to be managed, treated, or cured and advantageously spare a person at least some of the detriment associated with serious illness or premature death. (FDA 2009)

Agencies responsible for public health in the United States, such as the Agency for Healthcare Research and Quality (U.S. Preventive Services Task Force), the FDA, the American Cancer Society, and the Environmental Protection Agency, as well as national medical and professional societies

(American College of Radiology, the American College of Cardiology/ American Heart Association, the American Association of Physicists in Medicine, the Health Physics Society, and the American Medical Association) do not recommend general whole-body CT screening. The states of Texas and Pennsylvania have banned whole-body CT scans for general population screening, and other states are considering similar legislation.

The popularity of whole-body CT scanning for tumors extends worldwide in the industrial nations. Similar skepticism abounds about the usefulness of the technology for screening the general population. For example, the Department of Environment, Climate Change and Water of the New South Wales government in Australia cautions that when deciding whether to undergo a whole-body CT scan you should consider the following:

- The scan should only be undertaken as part of a comprehensive evaluation, including a physical examination, medical history and other tests.
- You should not undergo such a test without a written request from an independent medical practitioner.
- Whole-body scanning is not recommended for people under fifty years as they are more at risk of developing cancers as a result of this procedure.
- You should understand the risks involved and the scale of the radiation dose you will receive. These should be clearly explained to you by a medical practitioner.
- You should be asked to give your informed consent in writing prior to undergoing the whole-body CT scanning procedure.
- Choose a radiologist who specializes in CT imaging. The radiologist should also communicate with your medical practitioner.
- Choose a facility that is affiliated with a major health center. These providers are more likely to have high standards in terms of staff and equipment.
- Choose a practice with only the most up-to-date and best equipment. The best equipment is the multidetector CT with three-dimensional reconstructions. Other CT scanners that are also appropriate include the spiral or helical scanner and electron beam CT.
- Patients should be aware that other specific procedures are required in the case of virtual colonoscopy and certain other applications, such as evaluation of the coronary arteries for calcium deposits.
- In some examinations such as for abdominal (but not chest) scans, a contrast medium should also be used. This helps to differentiate between normal and abnormal tissues. Without the use of a contrast

medium, small lesions of the liver, kidneys, and pancreas may be missed, and any lesions that are detected may not be fully characterized. Discuss with your referring doctor if a contrast medium is required.

- Appropriate patient preparation should be performed for the organ being investigated (e.g., clearing of bowel contents for best results in virtual endoscopy). Check with your referring doctor as to what preparation is required (New South Wales Government Department of Environment 2008).

CHAPTER 15

Cost-Benefit of Medical Imaging

The ability to observe structure and function within the intact human body is a technological wonder unimaginable before the beginning of the twentieth century. In the twenty-first century, it would be unthinkable for many people in the industrial world to do without, particularly given the fact that most people have progressed beyond philosophical issues of personal boundaries (Kevles 1997, 1998). The value of the information gained from the technology is in improving patient outcome and quality of life. However, the magnitude of the increment in improvement provided by succeeding generations of technology is increasingly being scrutinized by people and the institutions responsible for paying the cost of the procedures.

While modern medical imaging technology provides unprecedented diagnostic capabilities, creating a tremendous demand for those services, the expenses associated with medical imaging have been rising exponentially. Greatly outstripping the increases in general clinical diagnostic testing, medical imaging costs are the fastest growing of high technology medical expenses. The Government Accountability Office released a report in June 2008 that corroborated a 2005 Medicare Payment Advisory Commission's study that pointed to high-tech imaging as the fastest growing component of physician's services paid for by Medicare. Increases in the proportion of nonhospital independent facilities and physician offices were particularly notable.

The recommended cost control remedy was requiring prior approval by the payer. While this seems like a logical control step, the American College of Radiologists supports an alternative criterion, an appropriateness determination, which, not surprisingly, focuses on the benefit of the medical imaging decided by the physician and the patient rather than

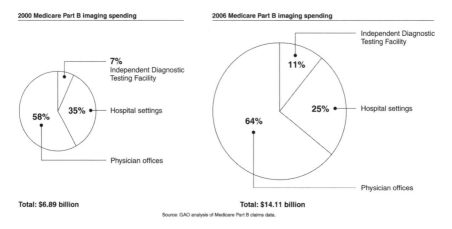

Figure 15.1 Medicare Part B spending on imaging by setting, 2000 and 2006. (Government Accountability Office.)

relying on radiology benefits managers who they feel are less tuned in to the medical need. Herein lays the controversy for medical imaging: the reconciliation of cost and access for patients.

One of the reasons for the increasing health care utilization and cost are the changing demographics in the industrial and developing world. The leading cause of death in the United States in 2005 for all ages under forty-five was accidents. Between the ages of forty-five and sixty-four cancer takes over as the leading cause, and for those sixty-five years of age and older, heart disease rises to the top, although malignancies continue to take a heavy toll, closely followed by cardio-vascular conditions (National Center for Health Statistics 2008, Table 31). However, the incidence of illness is not evenly distributed throughout the lifespan. In the industrial nations, it increases with age.

Figure 15.2 shows the distribution of usage of Medicare-paid medical imaging services in the United States by state. Not surprisingly, states with concentrations of older residents such as Florida and Arizona have higher expenditures.

Information compiled by the United Nations indicates that by the year 2050, 25 to 29 percent of the United States population will be over the age of sixty. The U.S. Centers for Disease Control and Prevention projects that 10 percent of the U.S. population, or more than 40 million people, will be seventy-five years or older by 2050 (National Center for Health Statistics 2008).

Canada, China, Russia, and countries in Europe are projecting more than 30 percent of their populations will be seventy-five years or older by then. On the other end of the spectrum, the majority of countries in Africa

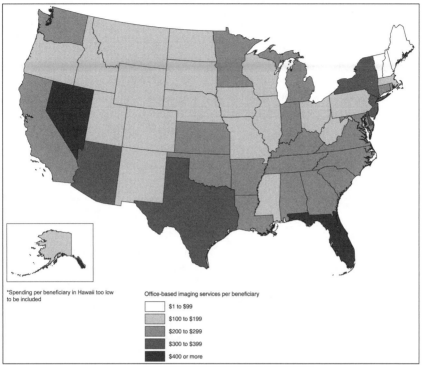

*Spending per beneficiary in Hawaii too low to be included

Office-based imaging services per beneficiary

	$1 to $99
	$100 to $199
	$200 to $299
	$300 to $399
	$400 or more

Sources: GAO analysis of Medicare Part B claims data, Map Resources (map).

Figure 15.2 The distribution of usage of Medicare-paid medical imaging services in the U.S. by state. (Government Accountability Office.)

are expected to have less than 19 percent in the boomer generation in their burgeoning populations. Since approximately 80 percent of illness in industrial nations occurs in the last 20 percent of life (Medical Imaging Technology Roadmap Steering Committee 2000), it is not difficult to deduce that the industrial nations will find their health care systems challenged, both with respect to their capacity for health care delivery and with their ability to pay for that health care. Medical imaging technology is seen as both a potential savior and demon. Cost increases in the technology beyond that in other areas threaten financial hardship for patients and ruin upon the whole health care system.

COST-BENEFIT ANALYSIS

The only fully justified reason for the use of an expensive technology such as medical imaging is that it will improve patient care and outcome at a reasonable economic cost to the individual and the society. The benefits come in a variety of shapes and sizes: (1) to the individual from more personalized medicine with individualized treatment because of earlier detection of subclinical disease, including better follow-up and understanding of the effect of treatment on the pathological process and less time out of life and work; (2) to patients in general by screening of a population or targeted subpopulation and a better assessment of risk factors and opportunities for disease prevention leading to decreased mortality and morbidity; and (3) to the health care enterprise for more rapid and accurate diagnosis, less time to the most effective treatment, shorter hospital stays, reduced need for long-term nursing, image-guided interventions, and effective use of expensive diagnostic and surgical equipment and facilities. The question is, in practice, how well is this being accomplished and at what cost.

Analyses of this type are difficult and controversial when applied to human life and suffering because they force evaluating a monetary expenditure against a valuation of life and the quality of that life extended by an intervention. It is less onerous and more straightforward to calculate whether the cost of a machine that makes doughnuts is less than the income from the sale of doughnuts that it produces before it needs to be replaced. Just what value should be placed on that extra five years of life given to a cancer survivor whose malignancy was picked up early by medical imaging? For an individual patient or their relative, there is no need to discuss the value, but for cost- and resource-constrained government and health care systems, it is an issue they increasingly have to deal with.

The terminology used by evaluators signals their difficulty in defining value for health care outcome. A traditional **Cost-benefit Analysis** of medical imaging or other interventions, which evaluates cost against the utility of the procedure, adjusted for pain and inconvenience, is not considered appropriate for ethical reasons because it puts a monetary value on life. **Cost-effective Analysis** is defined as gain in health compared with the cost of obtaining that gain. Gain here is most commonly measured in years of life added, or more specifically, quality-adjusted years of life gained. This is an attempt to account in some way for whether the extra year of living allows some form of return to a relatively normal life, at least not pain-filled or in a coma, and so on. For diagnosis, the criterion is the cost per correct diagnosis, although it does not necessarily include how valuable the diagnosis was. Some evaluators use **Cost-utility Analysis,** which adjusts for the "value attached to the benefits." This would encompass both patient and health care provider assessments of value. Other measures of effectiveness with less ethical baggage are lives saved, disability days lost or disability days avoided, cases detected, cases correctly staged (disease stage), and healthy years added.

Third-party payers (insurance companies and so on) and the government (Medicare) use some version of these analyses to set standards of what they will pay for. It is not completely clear in each case how the thresholds were determined. Originally, any new test was considered experimental and not reimbursed. After extensive use established clear benefits, particular tests could no longer reasonably be termed experimental. Payers were pressured or legislated into accepting responsibility for covering a proportion or all of those costs. This established a standard against which other tests could be compared. When new modalities came online, the avenue to certification was based on being as useful or having a comparable cost-benefit ratio to an established test. The same analysis is used to assess treatments for disease or surgeries (pathological or restorative). A standard or threshold for this ratio, also known as willingness-to-pay, averages around $50,000 per quality-adjusted life year (**QALY**). This consensus figure can be $20,000, $50,000, or $100,000 per QALY depending on the testing modality or therapeutic intervention (Valk et al. 2003, 796).

Table 15.1 Medicare Physician Fees for Most Commonly Billed Imaging Services in 2006, by Imaging Modality

Imaging modality	Most commonly billed imaging test	Fee for performing test	Fee for interpreting test	Total fee
MRI	MRI brain with and without dye	$995	$123	$1,118
Nuclear medicine	Heart image (3D) multiple	$471	$77	$548
CT	CT of head/brain without contrast	$189	$44	$233
Ultrasound	Doppler echo exam, heart	$69	$20	$90
X-ray and other std imaging	Chest X-ray	$19	$9	$28
Procedures using imaging	Injection for coronary X-ray	*	*	*

*Physician fee schedule does not include separate fees for this activity (e.g., surgery).

CONTROLLING COSTS

Medical imaging has grown to a greater than $100 billion per year business in the United States (Inglehart 2006). The combination of increasingly powerful but also progressively more expensive imaging technologies, increased use by physicians, and amplified expectations of patients that the latest technology be used to diagnose their condition drive the increases. In 1996, the U.S. Panel on Cost-effectiveness in Health and Medicine convened by the U.S. Public Health Service listed recommendations for performing and reporting cost-effect analyses of testing and medical procedures (Weinstein et al. 1996). In an attempt to control spending on imaging, the Deficit Reduction Act of 2005 (DRA 2005) capped Medicare payments on nonhospital imaging and computer-assisted imaging for the technical component at 2005 levels by limiting charges at a hospital to the lowest scale of cost charged by that hospital (Moser 2006).

DRA 2005 specifically targeted MRI, CT, X-rays, nuclear medicine (PET, SPECT), ultrasound, and bone densitometry. Only mammography was exempt from the cap. The cap primarily affected imaging in physician's offices and outpatient imaging facilities located outside of hospitals. Obtaining multiple images at the same time, even for medically indicated procedures, was discouraged by reducing payments by 25 percent in 2006 and by 50 percent thereafter. The reductions were greatest for MRI (34 percent), the most expensive of procedures, averaging 14 percent for all the other modalities. The federal budget calculates the accrued savings as a reduction in expense.

Radiologists have two main disagreements with this legislation. First, they feel that service providers have been singled out to bear the bulk of the cuts while little was being done to control the amount of testing being ordered, which they feel is the driving force for the increase in Medicare costs. Second, they feel that the criteria used to set reimbursements were inappropriate ("a blunt instrument") for situations outside of hospitals that have different abilities to distribute expenses and absorb costs of upgrading instrumentation. Not surprisingly, radiologists prefer the Medicare Fee for Service metric, which takes into account physician involvement and expenses as well as mandating a sustainable growth rate. A pay-for-performance schedule to control costs, such as have been established for other medical specialties, is being developed, but the specific requirements for imaging are still being worked out.

A study requested by Congress on the costs of medical imaging covering the period 2000–2006 was carried out by the U.S. Government

Table 15.2 Medicare Spending on Imaging Services Paid For Under the Physician Fee Schedule by Modality, 2000 through 2006.

Dollars (in millions) Imaging Modalities	Year						
	2000	2001	2002	2003	2004	2005	2006
CT	975	1,205	1,306	1,521	1,818	2,076	2,171
MRI	1,002	1,316	1,451	1,768	2,155	2,738	2,982
Nuclear Medicine	972	1,263	1,439	1,735	2,060	2,303	2,418
Ultrasound	1,842	2,116	2,204	2,490	2,823	3,208	3,334
X-rays and other standard imaging	1,711	1,925	2,013	2,189	2,391	2,464	2,485
Procedures that use imaging	386	473	555	686	840	708	715
Total for advanced imaging*	2,951	3,783	4,197	5,025	6,062	7,116	7,571
Total for standard imaging**	3,939	4,515	4,771	5,366	6,064	6,380	6,534
Overall total	6,891	8,298	8,969	10,390	12,106	13,496	14,105

*Advanced imaging includes MRI, nuclear medicine, and CT.
**Standard imaging included ultrasound, X-ray, and other standard imaging, and procedures that use imaging (surgery).

Accountability Office (GAO) (U.S. GAO 2008) and was published in 2008. It documented in detail the continuing expansion of the medical imaging enterprise and cost to Medicaid that led to DRA 2005. Those in opposition to the legislation condemned the haste in which DRA 2005 was drafted and enacted. They were concerned because it was felt that the developers of that legislation did not fully consider the ramifications to the medical community, manufacturers, or the patients they serve. Organizations such as the Access to Medical Imaging Coalition (AMIC), with constituents drawn from manufacturing, radiologists, physicians, and concerned patients, were created to address the DRA 2005 imaging cuts. They pushed for corrective legislation to suspend the DRA 2005-mandated cuts.

On May 8, 2007, Sen. Jay Rockefeller (D-W.Va.) and Gordon H. Smith (R-Ore.) introduced the bipartisan bill Access to Medicare Imaging Act of 2007 (S. 1338), calling for a two-year moratorium of the imaging cuts that went into effect the first of the year as a result of DRA 2005. Senator Rockefeller commented: "We are very concerned that patients who depend upon imaging services outside of the hospital setting, especially those patients in rural and underserved areas, will be particularly hard hit." Senator Smith spoke against the lack of consideration for the consequences of the deficit reduction legislation.

> Given the haste in which the DRA'05 legislation was crafted, it is imperative that we institute a two year delay to allow enough time for a thorough analysis by the Government Accountability Office (GAO). We should have a better understanding of the complexities and impacts brought about by these cuts before moving forward with a potentially damaging policy.

Similar legislation had been introduced in the House by Representatives Carolyn McCarthy (D-N.Y.), Joseph Pitts (R-Pa.), and Gene Green (D-Tex.) in April 2007.

Opponents of DRA 2005 feel that outpatient services curtailed by economics force the primarily elderly patients either to use overwhelmed hospital imaging centers or, lacking local facilities, to forgo diagnostic imaging altogether, showing up later with advanced cancers or other consequences that could have been forestalled by early diagnostic imaging. Dr. Steven A. Artz, professor of medicine, West Virginia University College of Medicine and chair of the West Virginia Chapter of the American Association of Clinical Endocrinologists (AACE) commented on the cuts on patient care.

> Medicare cuts to diagnostic imaging services have caused payments to go far below the costs to provide these procedures. A local community

Women's Health Clinic in Charleston has stopped performing osteoporosis screening and treatment services altogether because they can no longer afford to do the procedures. Our University practice in Charleston is concerned about whether we can handle the influx of elderly patients for these services and if patients will travel across town to our facility.

What remains is a complex scenario. The goal is to find equitable ways to control the escalating costs of medical imaging procedures while guaranteeing the delivery of sufficiently high-quality diagnostic information to provide for adequate medical care across the population throughout the country. The difficulty will be in balancing the economic resources with the needs and expectations of imaging providers and interpreters, patient care physicians, and the patient whose health is at stake.

CHAPTER 16

Accessibility of Medical Imaging in Developing Countries

In the United States and other industrial nations, we have taken medical imaging technology for granted almost since X-rays were first discovered and their remarkable penetrating qualities recognized by Roentgen at the end of the nineteenth century. Several generations have now grown up not knowing what it was like to be unsure about a broken bone or fear that a persistent cough was a harbinger of the dreaded "consumption" (tuberculosis). A couple's first baby picture is frequently an ultrasonogram, and they can find out whether their soon-to-be-born child is a boy or a girl. These simple procedures and the fantastically more sophisticated CAT scans, MRIs, and PET and SPECT scans are available to aid physicians to diagnose, plan surgeries, and measure organ function in or near most major population centers. Trained certified technicians operate well-maintained modern equipment digitally integrated with the scanners that are connected to secure patient information management systems. Health care systems with all of their caveats, backed up to various degrees by governments, provide patient access and a reasonable measure of financial support.

Contrast this to the situation in developing nations, particularly those in Africa. The World Health Organization (WHO) estimates that three-quarters of the world's population have no access to diagnostic imaging equipment such as radiology, ultrasound, magnetic resonance, and nuclear medicine (SPECT, PET) technologies (WHO 2003). WHO also estimates that 80 to 90 percent of diagnostic problems can be addressed easily by basic X-ray examination that does not include tomographic scanners, or by ultrasound. Two-thirds of the world's population is believed to not have access to even this minimal level of diagnostic technology (WHO 2009). It is easy to assign this disparity simply to a lack of economic resources given the state of developing nation economies; however, the difficulty is more deep-seated. Generally, equipment is lacking, and more than half of the equipment available is nonfunctional because of the lack of a reliable uninterrupted and stable power supply, improper maintenance, no spare parts, and a scarcity of trained and knowledgeable instrument repair technicians. Fourteen countries in Africa do not have a single radiologist (Hoaglin et al. 2006, 12). Ironically, often what equipment is available is too sophisticated for the application, and health care personnel do not know how to use it.

The mismatch between the requirements of the diagnostic facilities and the available equipment is fed by the fact that 95 percent of medical imaging technology is imported from the industrial countries that possess the technology and manufacturing capacity to produce the equipment and achieve an economy of scale. Local industries have not developed or cannot compete. Multiple programs sponsored by non-governmental organizations such as the World Health Imaging Alliance (http://www.worldhealthimaging.org) donate medical imaging equipment to developing nations. Particularly in the case of used equipment, it may be outmoded and frequently is not compatible with other systems in its new home. Additional factors come into play that compound the impact of the well-intentioned donations. Diagnostic imaging competes in the government health care arena with the more basic need of the population for safe, clean water and adequate nutrition. As a result, the basic infrastructure for delivery and support of imaging services has languished. Often the procedures for planning and building the required infrastructure are obscure as are the mechanisms for evaluation and acquisition of expensive technical equipment. Even the information essential for determining just what resources are available to make an informed decision about what needs to be done and what can be done is not available or is of questionable validity. Even in countries where the economic circumstances are favorable, medical diagnostic imaging often flounders.

Habib Zaidi from the Division of Nuclear Medicine of the Geneva University Hospital in Switzerland places the onus for the problem on a lack of infrastructure, which is brought about by a failure to recognize the importance for a developing country to establish the requisite standards of training, maintenance, safety, and data handling (Zaidi 2008). Most developing countries rely on the industrial countries for advanced education and training, which is implicitly coordinated with the industrial nation's standards and common resources. When the medical physicists and others return to their home country, the standards are different or nonexistent. Additionally, the assumptions about such resources as routine maintenance, spare parts, service contracts, or even a stable constant electrical supply no longer apply. The whole medical system is less computerized from the equipment to the lack of standardized electronic patient recordkeeping. This makes delivering the available diagnostic imaging data and its interpretation to the physician in time for it to be incorporated into the patient's treatment plan difficult and of reduced value to the patient. Physicians in such circumstances learn to do without this sometimes-critical piece of information that can make the difference between the right and wrong diagnosis and result in a misguided treatment plan.

Besides the handicaps of inadequately maintained high-tech equipment, equipment that functional often is not properly matched with a data processing and analysis system; additionally, numbers of adequately trained medical physicists or radiologists are insufficient to process the data or interpret the final images, respectively. In the short term at least, some stopgap solutions have been proposed. Rotary International and the World Health Imaging Alliance (WHIA), a nonprofit organization (http://www.worldhealthimaging.org), organizes the "funding, deployment, training and servicing" of digital X-ray systems through a network of collaborator organizations (WHIA 2009).

They address the issue of outmoded equipment, when possible, by retrofitting analog systems by replacing film with a robust solid-state phosphor screen read with a computed radiography reader device to generate quality digital data. Importantly, they focus on sustainability of the imaging site and maintaining compliance with international standards. A WHO-approved X-ray machine manufactured by Sedecal Global is mated with a digital medical imaging system provided by Carestream Health, a medical and dental imaging and information technology company, operated with software systems by Merge Healthcare. A WHIA Box integrates the essential electronic technologies that can be used in the uncontrolled and frequently hostile conditions. These include touchscreen environment-resistant computing, cellular and wireless connectivity, global positioning system (GPS) tracking, and a biometric reader (no passwords). To address the general lack of recordkeeping in remote clinical sites, electronic records are compatible with international standards, including usage tracking and accountability. Electronic medical records and personal health records can be maintained in this portable box. Because trained radiologists are at a premium and frequently not present at the clinical site, this system is designed to take advantage of teleradiology and telemedicine applications, allowing data acquired at outlying sites to be transmitted to central facilities for analysis and interpretation. An Internet-based WHIA Web portal for data is under development. The ability to interface the WHIA system is being tested with a variety of film-based diagnostic X-ray instrumentation used in community health care clinics in the Western Cape of South Africa. Less comprehensively integrated data transmittal systems for teleradiology that would use remote image production from a digital data stream have been proposed using digital cellular phone technology (Granot, Ivorra, and Rubinsky 2008), although some technical issues related to current cellular phone technology may need to be addressed before this becomes feasible.

Government programs frequently are unable to provide adequate access for their populations to medical imaging. Medical imaging facilities along with other high-tech resources often end up in the capital cities, for a variety of reasons. Many people cannot afford to travel for diagnosis and treatment. Private enterprise sometimes tries to fill the need. The capacity of such facilities generally is not up to the task, and the cost is beyond the means of the majority of the population. Adding to this an assortment of socioeconomic factors and cultural biases further reduces or even flatly denies care to certain individuals. Zaidi feels that effectively utilizing the resources available in a given country is more important than obtaining additional resources, upgrading to state-of-the-art equipment, or campaigning for more resources. The effectiveness depends more directly on adequately educating and training operating and maintenance personnel. In addition, advocating the use of standard diagnostic methods and therapeutic approaches by physicians will provide greater benefits to patients than high-tech instrumentation.

CHAPTER 17

Admissibility of Medical Images as Evidence in a Court of Law

X-RAYS IN COURT

The first use of medical imaging technology as evidence in a court of law came within a month of Roentgen's announcement of his discovery of X-rays. The ghostly picture of Frau Roentgen's hand with a finger encircled by the dark band of her wedding ring on the front page of the Vienna newspaper *Neue Freie Presse* advertised the utility of the mysterious rays to detect metal objects. Around the same time Roentgen was making sure of his observations, December 1895, Tolman Cunnings, a young Canadian, was involved in a Montreal barroom altercation and was shot in the leg. Surgeons at General Hospital in the city were unable to find the bullet and decided to leave it alone. Cunnings filed suit in February 1896 against his alleged assailant, and his attorney announced that "Professor Roentgen's new photographic discovery will be used in evidence" (Brecher and Brecher 1969, 19). An X-ray photograph of Cunnings's leg made by a physicist at McGill University in Montreal located the missing bullet. Cunnings's physician used the picture to guide surgical removal of the object, which was causing his patient considerable pain. Cunnings's attorney used the bullet and the radiograph of the bullet inside his client's leg to obtain a swift conviction a mere two months after the discovery of X-rays. X-ray evidence soon was used to reconstruct criminal acts, such as corroborating testimony determining the angle from which a gun had been fired.

In mid-summer 1896, a U.S. case involving X-ray images as evidence was brought in Denver, Colorado. James Smith had fallen off a ladder that April, sustaining an impacted fracture of the head of his femur and, after examination by a prominent surgeon, had been diagnosed with a contusion. Several months later, with the pain in his hip unabated, Smith had his hip X-rayed, which showed the fracture. The subsequent trial focused squarely on whether X-rays could be admitted as evidence in a case similar to fingerprints or bullet matching to a firearm. Both sides were aware that this case could set a U.S. jurisprudential precedent. They agreed that an X-ray photograph was not the same as a regular photograph, which could not see beneath the skin. Already, several U.S. judges had refused to accept X-ray radiographs as evidence "because there is no proof that such a thing is possible. It is like offering the photograph of a ghost where there is no proof that there is any such thing as a ghost" (Withers 1931). No one had actually seen the living broken bone. Smith's lawyers provided a series of demonstrations, including X-rays of objects such as a clock showing the internal mechanism with which the judge and jury were familiar, and then showed an X-ray of a normal femur followed by an X-ray of the damaged femur. Smith won his case, and in doing so established the credibility of X-ray evidence in court.

X-ray evidence soon was used for forensics in serving the dead as well as the living. Dentists rapidly saw the value of X-ray images. The enamel on teeth absorbs even more X-rays than bone and cavities and malformations were obvious on the plates. Personal dental history was unique to the individual. Thus, dentists accumulated the first archives of medical imaging records that could identify individuals even after death. Dental records and X-rays are important tools for modern coroners. The first recorded use of X-rays to identify the dead was in the aftermath of a fire at a benefit bazaar in Paris, France, on May 4, 1897, in which more than two hundred socially prominent patrons died. X-rays were used to identify the bodies that were charred beyond recognition.

One of the issues that X-ray images created was that, unlike regular photographs that the general public or a jury could interpret, X-ray images require specialized knowledge and experience to interpret the shades of gray. This was particularly true for the early radiograms, which suffered from scattered radiation and weak or variable X-ray sources, resulting in poor contrast and foggy images. When dealing with complex technologies, a familiar solution is to have an expert witness interpret data that the average jury member would have no reason to be familiar with. This expert witness can testify to the quality and authenticity of the information and provide some kind of statement about what is being shown. At the time X-rays were being introduced as evidence, however, a backlash was cresting against the excesses of disagreements during expert testimony in court cases, particularly those involving medical malpractice, spurring calls for reform from both the legal and medical sides. X-ray image were initially considered another form of photograph and hence could be admitted as illustrative evidence. The image could be used by an expert to demonstrate a point, but he could not say what the image showed. Human testimony was required to validate the image. Interpreting the image was left up to the jury. The problem was that whatever the X-ray showed was hidden from the naked human eye, so how could someone, even an expert witness, vouch for what was normally invisible. Judge Le Fevre in the Colorado James Smith case sidestepped the issue by admitting the evidence on the basis that the process that produced it was known to be reliable (Golan 2004). Several X-ray pictures taken of the same broken bone produced the same image.

The Tennessee Supreme Court in 1897 stated that, "New as this process is, experiments made by scientific men, as shown by this record, have demonstrated its power to reveal to the natural eye the understructure of the human body, and that its various parts can be photographed as its exterior surface has been and now is" (*Bruce v. Beall* 1897, 99 Tenn. 303, 41 S.W. 445). With the weight of a state supreme court behind this interpretation, other states soon followed suit, including Maine in 1899; Massachusetts, Wisconsin, and Washington, D.C., in 1901; and Nebraska, Illinois, and Arkansas over the next four years.

By 1900, only four years after their discovery, the quality and reproducibility of X-ray imaging had improved dramatically, and a body of literature of those images was accumulating along with a growing group of physicians who now had considerable experience in interpreting the images. The American Roentgen Ray Society, founded that year, worked to have radiology accepted as a specialized medical profession in its own right. The first X-ray images were taken by all sorts of people. The equipment was simple even though no one really understood the true nature of X-rays or recognized the delayed dangers that would claim the appendages and lives of those who worked with this mysterious invisible light. Anyone with a Crookes tube, a film cassette, and a photographic darkroom could hang out a shingle. In addition, the equipment was notoriously fickle. No two tubes generated the same amount of X-rays or X-rays with the same range of penetration, and even the same tube at different times of the day could be drastically different, hence, the wide variation in the images. The Roentgen Society sought to professionalize the process, making it a distinct medical profession with common standards of education, training, ethics, and competence. They also separated the process of creating the image, which was a technical process that with the improved equipment on the market could be achieved by many nonmedical personnel, from the interpretation of the image. Reading the images required a great deal of training, experience, and a medical background in anatomy and pathology. The field of radiology developed over the first two decades of the twentieth century, providing experts to interpret the X-ray images. An uneasy truce between the legal and medical professions over the admission of X-ray images as evidence permits expert testimony from radiologists. Similar battles have occurred for other forms of visual presentation that cannot be vouched for by direct human experience and periodically erupt anew.

The traditional X-ray is an absorption image, a shadow, or skiagraph as they were known in the early days. A fluoroscope substituted a glowing fluorescent screen for the film. The bones of the hand cast a shadow much like the flesh-covered hand cast a shadow in sunlight. It was not too difficult a stretch to appreciate the similarities. Then technology intervened to create three-dimensional images from a series of "slices," tomography. Early tomographic methods used controlled movement of either the subject or the X-ray source and the film to generate a sharp image at the center of rotation while blurring the background. This was like creating a sharp image of a racehorse by panning along with the horse and smearing the background.

These images could be appreciated by most people. Even before rudimentary computers, physicists realized that mathematical manipulation of the X-ray intensities collected during the scans could produce even higher quality images. These computations, however, were not intuitive operations that any juror could perform in his or her head. In terms of the legal rationale, this required a further extension of faith that the mathematical transformation was yielding a true image rather than a series of artifacts. As the medical imaging technologies moved further and further afield from human physical senses, the more reluctant has been the jurisprudential establishment to accept the output at face value. Where information from these types of imaging has been allowed, courts have had to rely increasingly heavily on expert witness testimony.

Structure-based medical imaging technologies (CT, MRI) have been more readily accepted as evidence than the functional imaging technologies (fMRI, PET, SPECT) when presented appropriately by a properly credentialed expert witness. The sheer volume of CT and MRI images used in diagnostic medicine and the consistency and reliability of the technologies in producing structural images of the brain have lead to their ready acceptance for reporting structure accurately. What remains at issue, as with all types of medical imaging, is the connection between alterations in the observed structure and the interpretation as to the meaning of those differences (Moriarty 2008). What is normal, or what deviates from normality but is benign versus what is truly pathological? The data collected on a large number of individuals have provided some definition of the scope of interpersonal variation that an expert witness can use to make his or her interpretation.

The newer forms of imaging, fMRI, PET, and SPECT, open up a whole new dimension. These technologies do not visualize structure per se. They report on functional properties of regions of tissues or organs that may or may not, depending on the particular property being detected, correspond to a specific physical structure. For diagnostic and therapeutic purposes combined with other information, this may provide sufficient information to support a treatment plan or to warrant further testing of additional parameters. For evidentiary purposes in a malpractice case, however, the specificity of the functional changes for the condition and the reliability of the method to consistently document those changes become the issue. This is much more difficult to prove. There can be multiple causes that produce a particular functional signal, some of which are normal physiological conditions and others that are part of normal biological variation between individuals. Further research is required to develop procedures and standards to sufficiently solidify the connection of function with the condition to be admissible as evidence in court. This may be achievable only for a subset of functional measurements, because in addition to practicality, certain functional measurements introduce questions of medical ethics (Moriarty 2008).

THE LIVING BRAIN IN COURT

X-rays were the leading edge of a wave of technological innovations that assailed the basic premises of jurisprudence, which was based on human testimony. Eyewitness testimony was the gold standard, although recent studies have shown that such testimony is accurate approximately half of the time. This rising amount of technical evidence demanded a set of standards as to which types of evidence would be admissible. A U.S. Court of Appeals ruling in 1923 for the District of Columbia Circuit (*United States v. Frye* 293F.1013 D. C. Cir. 1923) established the Frye Test, which among other things required "general acceptance in the relevant scientific community."

More than the passage of time after the invention of new technology is required for this acceptance. The first introduction of forensic DNA analysis as evidence, now used to identify individuals from their genotype, occurred in 1986 in a United Kingdom immigration case. It required statistical analyses and a consensus of expert testimony to establish its credibility in the forensic and genetic science communities. Data from several current medical imaging modalities, despite being invented and practiced for many years, do not yet meet the Frye criteria to be introduced as evidence in a court of law. They are informative for medical diagnosis and treatment, often figuring in life and death decisions for patients, but the interpretation of those data has not yet reached the threshold of general acceptance in the scientific community.

The issue became more complicated when in 1993 the U.S. Supreme Court decided that the Federal Rules of Evidence drafted in 1942 should take precedence over the Frye Test. This case (*Daubert v. Merrill Dow Pharmaceuticals, Inc.* 113 S. Ct. 2786, 1993) became known as the Daubert Rule and is now the current standard for scientific testimony. Other cases decided by the Supreme Court (*General Electric Co. v. Joiner*, 522 U.S. 136, 1997; *Kumho Tire Co., Ltd. v. Carmichael,* 526 U.S. 137, 1999) also have influenced the admission of expert evidence. Whereas the Frye Test relied on the scientific community to determine whether a given technology or method demonstrated reliability and was considered "generally acceptable," Daubert made the presiding judge, who rarely had any scientific or medical training, solely responsible for determining what scientific testimony to admit based on what she or he deemed "relevant" and "reliable." Conclusions based on the method had to be testable compared with a different accepted method, an error rate had to be established, and the method had to be one that was generally accepted by scientists and the medical community as demonstrated by peer-reviewed publications. Further explication (*Anonymous Daubert v. Merrill Dow Pharmaceuticals, Inc.* 509 U.S. 579, 597, 1993, 2005) concluded that such expert testimony had to meet two additional standards. First, it had to "fit"—have "a valid scientific connection to the pertinent inquiry" and be "sufficiently tied to the facts of the case that will aid the jury in resolving factual dispute." Second, it must have "weight"—a sufficient degree of importance to influence the court's judgment in the case. Considerable discussion has centered on whether this change in the rules of engagement has resulted in the admission of more "junk science" into evidence as a result of judges taking a gatekeeper role in deciding which expert testimony would be allowed for a particular trial (Kulich, Maciewicz, and Scrivani 2009). Interestingly, this and other interpretations of Federal Rules of Evidence are only binding for *federal* courts. State courts and state legislatures usually follow along, but they are by no means required to do so.

An Example of a Direct Forensic Application of a Medical Imaging Technology: Lie Detection

The human capability for deception is a trait of much concern in a court of law. Who is telling the truth and who is lying? As discussed, the cornerstone of evidence verification in the legal system is the requirement for a human to vouch for its veracity, the human witness. Deception is believed to be inherent in humans (Vrij 2001). Fortunately, the trait is not well developed in most individuals (Etcoff 2000), which allows society and the courts to function. In some instances, technological means have been sought to verify the truth of testimony. Determining the absolute truth of a statement by an individual in a completely objective manner is a difficult thing to accomplish, impossible according to some critics. The neurophysiological basis for deception is incompletely understood. The current standard is the polygraph technique, invented in 1921, which monitors certain physiological reactions mediated by the peripheral nervous system: skin conductance, blood pressure, perspiration, and breathing patterns. The responses of these parameters are monitored under controlled conditions during a standard mode of questioning, usually forced-choice in which the subject selects from a set of answers about the case. In addition to technical and environmental difficulties, it is possible for a savvy subject to game the technology to produce an unreliable result. Certain mental conditions can produce spurious results. This reveals the fundamental issue that deception is a voluntary product of the CNS. Although the details are far from completely understood, the neurologic implementation of deception integrates the output of multiple brain regions before it is finally reflected in the responses of the peripheral nervous system. Thus, the basis of the current standard, the polygraph, is indirect and subject to interference. Polygraph evidence is admitted in court only under certain circumstances. New Mexico is the only state in which polygraph forensic lie detection is generally accepted. Despite these failings, the polygraph has been the gold standard against which other methods for determining truth and falsehood have been compared for almost a century.

Neuropsychologists have sought a method with a more solid foundation in brain function during thought processes. Electroencephalography (EEG), the recording of electrical potentials from the brain, measures brain electrical activity through a series of patch electrodes placed on areas of the scalp. This is an averaging technique that sums electrical fields generated by neuronal firings in superficial areas of the brain. Temporal and regional patterns of activity reveal neurophysiological events at the level of the

CNS. Activity patterns generated in response to the same or a similar standard questioning paradigm as that used for polygraph testing can be analyzed. It is feasible to distinguish between lie and truth under forced-choice questioning by this technique, under controlled laboratory conditions. EEG-based lie detection technology was developed in India where it has been used as evidence in court. The issue again is reliability, because some interpersonal variability as well as a number of medical conditions, some diagnosable and others not, can influence the results. A high degree of expertise is required to interpret the EEG results, which generates variability among evaluators.

fMRI, with its ability to localize areas of neuronal activity within the brain and the perceived safety of the technique, is an attractive methodology to differentiate lie from truth (Langelben 2008). The same question-and-answer testing is required as for the other methods. In fMRI, direct neural substrates are evaluated in situ and simultaneously without intervening layers of response, a more primal readout. Although specific brain areas are localized by the imaging, the BOLD fMRI measurements actually detect changes in blood flow to that brain region, not the electrical events. The blood flow changes are in response to increased neuronal requirements for oxygen and glucose when action potentials are being generated. The apparent directness of the measurement attracted the interest of neuropsychologists who were searching for a way to unambiguously identify activity in areas that signaled the lying brain. In laboratory experiments, stereotypic responses in certain areas were linked to lying. Accuracies for lie detection ranged between 76 and 90 percent (Kozel et al. 2005; Langelben et al. 2005). The hoped-for clarity remains to be achieved, however. In part, this is due to interpersonal brain differences, and in part due to interferences from activations occurring to other stimuli, real and imagined. Unfortunately, the method is still vulnerable to countermeasures. It turned out to be relatively easy to interfere with the relevant brain area activations, if the subject were so inclined. Continued study under controlled conditions may provide a sufficient database to allow forensic applications of the technology.

CHAPTER 18

Ethics of Medical Imaging

In the twenty-first century, the average person does not consider an X-ray of an injured arm to look for a broken bone an invasion of his or her personal space or an assault on the sanctity of the human body. It is so commonplace and the potential benefits so far outweigh the drawbacks that these concerns are rarely an issue. That would not have been true just a few centuries ago, and the relationship between the intact body and medical imaging still concerns philosophers, artists, and writers (Schinzel 2006). These cultural issues are considered in some detail in other forums (Chrysanthou 2002; Doby and Alker 1997; Kevles 1998; van Dijck 2005).

INDIVIDUALITY AND THE LIMITS OF PRIVACY

Within biological variation, structural parts of the human body are quite similar from one individual to the next. An arm is an arm, a heart is a heart, and a liver is a liver. Their functions are also fairly well understood. The brain is an organ of which we have a relatively rudimentary understanding. Concealed within a bony skull, anatomists, histologists, and neuroscientists have built up a map of the brain's physical structure and assigned functional roles to different regions based on what they learned from studies on other animals and from accidents, developmental disorders, disease, and medical interventions. Even with the contributions from noninvasive medical imaging technology, there is much that we do not know or understand of how the human brain works. In particular, we do not know how to account for distinctly human attributes that philosophers have defined, such as thought and self-knowledge. In Western cultures, the brain is considered to absolutely define the individual and is the seat of free will and moral judgment such as lying. Because of these supraphysiological functionalities, brain imaging poses unique ethical considerations, which have drawn attention from medical ethicists as well as from legal ethicists for whom structural or functional imaging is presented in evidence in courts of law.

By structural imaging (CT, MRI), within the scope of biological variation, normal brain structures are not remarkably different in any way that we can connect with performance. We know, however, that normal people have different personalities, they learn best by different modalities, and they respond to stimuli in different ways. Yet, we do not understand in any great detail the basis for these differences. The lack of knowledge is passed off by saying that individuals are simply "wired differently." Many neuroscientists believe that ultimately structural differences account for many of these differences, but resolving those differences is beyond our present capabilities. However, with further development of technology and perhaps discovery of new modalities of imaging, enough detail about neural connections and circuitry might permit the assignment of cause and effect. In diseases that affect neuronal development, as well as traumatic injuries, the "wiring" is clearly disturbed and neuronal tracts are disrupted, leading to profound functional deficits. Additionally, in more structurally subtle conditions, neurotransmitter systems or inhibitory or excitatory connections are out of balance, again causing disturbances in brain activity. The difficulty comes in connecting a difference in some parameter that can be monitored to a particular defect— that is, being able to say a given signal causes a specific consequence with high degree of reliability. This lack of certainty affects diagnostic and therapeutic decisions and has resulted in the exclusion of functional imaging information as evidence in a court of law.

A variety of functional imaging readouts have the potential to tease out some of the operational differences between function and dysfunction. Unfortunately, few are direct measures of brain function. Most also have low structural resolution. A functional image is quite different than a structural image. It does not necessarily correspond to a specific structure that can be visualized by eye or by nonvisible radiation structural imaging. It is an intrinsic signal (fMRI) or a compartment or region into which the imaging probe can penetrate (MRI contrast agent, PET, SPECT). When superimposed on structural images to give a sense of anatomical localization, functional images often appear to be floating in space, dissociated from their surroundings. This makes it difficult to reliably assign changes of intensity to particular physical causes.

Functional imaging has been a widely used research tool for studing the involvement of different brain areas in sensory processing and various mental efforts such as calculation, long- and short-term memory recall, language, decision making, and movement. Different areas of the brain "light up" as they are activated for the different tasks. The main regions activated are conserved between individuals, but additional regions are activated on a consistent basis within the same individual to accomplish a particular mental process that probably accounts for differences in how that person's brain handles a task. It is not always clear exactly how that brain region is contributing to the process, or whether it is involved at all. The human brain is often dealing with multiple inputs at the same time, even when best efforts are made to isolate extraneous stimuli.

The most commonly used functional imaging tools are blood flow and oxygenation monitored by fMRI, which uses the blood's own hemoglobin molecule as an endogenous probe, and ^{18}F-fluorodeoxyglucose (^{18}F-FDG), a PET imaging radiotracer, that labels cells using glucose as an energy source. These are powerful tools for monitoring function in a variety of tissues and organs—muscle, pancreas, and kidney. They are particularly useful for visualizing the activation of specific areas of the brain previously only monitored but not pinpointed by surface electrodes (EEG), or less frequently, direct insertion of electrodes into the brain. The patterns of oxygenated blood flow and metabolic activity, respectively, are interpreted as indicators of cellular activity, usually inferred to be neurotransmission. Conversely, disturbed or absent patterns are considered hallmarks of dysfunction, although the specific defect is not directly identified.

Persistent Vegetative State

In 1994, a Multi-Society Task Force established diagnostic criteria for brain injury resulting in a persistent vegetative state. They distinguished it from other stages of increasingly reduced consciousness; the locked-in state, stupor and obtundication, coma, and finally brain death, which involves the loss of all higher brain functions and all brain stem function, including reflexes. An individual such as Terri Schiavo, who was maintained after a hypoxic incident in a persistent vegetative state for fifteen years, shows no awareness of self or environment, no meaningful response to stimuli or interaction with others, and incontinence. Autonomic and brainstem function sufficient for sleep and wake cycles and survival is maintained along with variable cranial nerve and spinal reflexes. Some ten to twenty-five thousand adults and six to ten thousand children in the United States are in a persistent vegetative state (Perry, Churchill, and Kirschner 2005). One percent of those in a persistent vegetative state suffering a nontraumatic illness for more than three months achieve good recovery with moderate disability. *None* of those lingering in the condition for more than six months or those experiencing a traumatic injury resulting in a persistent vegetative state that lasts for a year have recovered.

Imaging methods can document the structural changes that have occurred in individuals in the different states of reduced consciousness and help support prognostic indications based on the observed damage to brain areas. For the persistent vegetative state, imaging can go beyond the dismal statistics by providing objective information on the severity of brain damage to help families with decisions on continued life support. In Terri Shiavo's case, an MRI could not be performed because of the previous implantation of a thalamic stimulator.

Privacy

The privacy of the individual is a jealously guarded right in the United States. From time to time, a national identity card for citizens has been proposed to replace the inconsistent state-run system and has been repeatedly and roundly defeated. In Europe, people wonder what the issue is for Americans. Protection of medical records, especially with increased exposure of records with electronic recordkeeping and telemedicine, although logical in order to avoid discrimination against individuals with health conditions for insurance, loans, or employment, has resulted in massive regulation and bureaucracy as well as the development of a considerable ethics industry.

For some people, the concept of privacy extends to the inside of the brain itself. What right does a medical practitioner, outside of a research study where informed consent has been sought and granted, have to observe brain region activation occurring outside of the specific regions being studied and consented? What if brain patterns, like genetics, could be associated with a tendency toward a mental illness such as schizophrenia, or toward violent or other socially unacceptable behavior, racism, criminal tendencies, liberalism, conservatism, and so on? Similar to genetic markers or even mutations, the brain activity patterns could not determine with certainty when or even if that behavior or tendency would manifest in the individual in which they were observed (Marano 2003). Genetic counseling is mandated when genetic testing is performed. Retaining records of brain activity observations, even without analysis, poses an ethical dilemma because linking currently uninterpretable brain activity patterns to medical conditions or mental health issues in the future could constitute improper use of medical records. Additionally, most likely this information would raise issues about whether the subject could give adequately informed consent. Adequate safeguards would be required to restrict access to this information. Under what conditions would it be legitimate for insurance companies, employers, spouses, or even parents to obtain this information?

The same issues exist for imaging the binding of radioligands for receptors in the brain or elsewhere. PET and SPECT radioligands can localize and quantify receptors, and can transport mechanisms, enzymes, and ion channels associated with cellular processes and pathways. These radioligands are most frequently used in research studies to understand how systems work rather than as diagnostic agents. The relative amounts of serotonin receptors versus dopamine receptors in specific brain regions can be determined to explain certain types of behavior. Information of this type could be misused in the same ways as the activity of brain regions.

Mind Reading

It is beyond current analytical capabilities to distinguish background brain activity from patterns that are related to the reason for performing the diagnostic or research imaging. The brain is a multilevel processor of information, so the potential exists for several activities to be running concurrently. Could some of these extra events be a person's private thoughts? Is it ethical for the imager to access these events that will be recorded along with the consented diagnostic information? To what use might such "mind reading" be put by government, police, and the military. Could evidence of this type be used in court?

Incidental Findings

When structural or functional brain scans are performed, a great deal of information is obtained that is not directly related to either the objectives of a research study employing imaging or to the condition for which a patient is being evaluated in diagnostic imaging. Unexpected masses, malformations, aneurisms, indications of current or past trauma, or anatomical evidence of dementia are observed with regularity, even in clinically normal individuals. This collateral information is termed "incidental findings." Incidental findings are defined as "observations of potential clinical significance unexpectedly discovered in healthy subjects or patients recruited to brain imaging research studies and unrelated to the purpose or variables of the study" (Illes et al. 2006). Most of these discoveries in medical imaging occur with MRI because it is more often used in normal populations and because it does not require exposure of normal individuals to ionizing radiation for which no benefit to the subject is expected from the procedure. MRI is more sensitive to small changes in the environment of the water molecules that make up its image.

A number of studies observed a prevalence of incidental findings during imaging of between 13 and 84 percent, depending on the study. Immediate referrals were made in 1.2 percent of the cases, urgent referrals in 1.8 to 43 percent, and no referrals in 40.4 percent of the cases (Wolf et al. 2008). This contrasts with studies that suggest that clinically significant and identifiable neuropathologies occur in 0.5 to 2 percent of the normal population. Data are scarce on the utility of brain imaging to screen asymptomatic individuals for clinically relevant pathologies. This is particularly true for the lower resolution nondiagnostic MRI and contrast MRI employed for collecting data in psychology or physiology research studies. These observations suggest that reporting of incidental findings constitute an ethical challenge to researchers and imagers.

The ethical concerns arise from whether a clinically normal subject should be informed of the detection of an apparent abnormality. The dramatic difference between the incidence of detection of clinically silent events and clinically significant events (13 to 84 percent versus 0.5 to 2 percent) suggests that much unnecessary angst and financial cost would be incurred by following up on all incidental findings. Additionally, a given research team may not have the necessary imaging and clinical expertise to make a judgment, particularly for nonmedical imaging studies that are not designed to detect clinically relevant changes. The informed consent agreements reached with subjects should spell out whether or not incidental findings will be reported to the individual. Assuming that no report means that no abnormalities were detected could be as damaging to a subject as reporting a clinically silent abnormality and could have legal repercussions.

Prior ethics arguments over the benefit of general medical screening and genetic screening support a subject's right *not* to know. Like genetic predisposition, a deviation from normal structure does not necessarily predict a clinical effect, nor does it indicate when it might manifest (Cho 2008). Protection of a subject's imaging record confidentiality needs to be maintained. Knowledge of prior existence of a medical condition could jeopardize future medical insurability. Future research may establish cause and effect between previously unrecognized connections that exist between abnormalities believed to be benign and clinical outcomes. These same issues have been addressed, and to date, legislation and a legal basis exist for maintaining confidentiality of genetic information.

CHAPTER 19

Mandatory Ultrasound Legislation

Abortion is a hot-button issue that has polarized and inflamed public opinion and politics for many years. Even with the legal hurdles and societal implications, more than 1 million pregnancies are terminated every year in the United States. This indicates that serious issues are driving demand for the procedure. It is not the purpose of this section to debate the pros and cons of the current state of abortion regulation in the United States, which at present is a protected right initiated by the historic *Roe vs. Wade* U.S. Supreme Court decision. Instead, it will address the mandatory use of medical imaging technology, specifically ultrasound imaging, for nonmedical purposes to satisfy a legal requirement of informed consent for an abortion to be performed.

This is the latest wrinkle introduced into the regulation of abortion over the past decade in many states. An ultrasound must be performed, the woman must be offered the opportunity to review the image(s), listen to a fetal heartbeat, be offered additional counseling, and given the opportunity to change her mind about proceeding with the abortion procedure. Although couched as a means to ensure that the woman's consent to the procedure is "fully informed," critics contend that the requirement is a thinly veiled attempt to emotionalize an already traumatic situation for a woman who has made a decision to terminate the pregnancy.

LEGISLATION OF MANDATORY ULTRASOUND BEFORE AN ABORTION

Although Sen. Sam Brownback (R-Kans.) introduced the Ultrasound Informed Consent Act in the U.S. Congress on September 20, 2007, no federal law requires ultrasound examination for an abortion. As of July 1, 2009, seven states required verbal communication or written materials, including information on obtaining no-cost ultrasound services, to be provided to a woman seeking an abortion, while thirteen regulate the provision of ultrasound services by the abortion provider.

The specifics vary from state to state. As an example quoted from current legislation, the key requirements for Texas are set forth in the Woman's Right to Know Act, amended May 1, 2009, by the Committee Substitute for Senate Bill (CSSB)182 to revise informed consent in Chapter 171 of the Health and Safety Code.

Under Health and Safety Code, ch. 171, the Woman's Right to Know Act, a person may not perform an abortion without the voluntary and informed consent of the woman on whom the abortion is to be performed. In order for consent to be considered informed and voluntary, the woman must be informed of:

1. the name of the physician who will perform the abortion
2. the risks associated with abortion and with carrying the child to term
3. the probable gestational age of the unborn child at the time the abortion is to be performed
4. available assistance for prenatal and neonatal care, and childbirth
5. the father's liability for child support
6. private agencies provide pregnancy prevention counseling and medical referrals; and
7. the woman's right to review printed materials provided by the Department of State Health Services.

Prior to the abortion, the woman must certify in writing that she received the above information, and the physician who is to perform the abortion must retain a copy of this certification. The information in the printed materials, the name of the physician who will perform the abortion, and the probable gestational age of the unborn child at the time the abortion is to be performed must be provided orally, by telephone, or in person, and at least 24 hours prior to performance of the abortion.

The information provided to the woman may not be conveyed by audio or video recording. The amendment adds:

Consent to an abortion was voluntary and informed only if the physician or the physician's agent:

1. provided the pregnant woman with the printed materials she currently has a right to review
2. informed her that she was not required to review those materials; and

3. provided her with a form entitled "Ultrasound Election" that stated "Texas law requires you to undergo an ultrasound prior to receiving an abortion," with space for the woman to elect whether or not to see and hear the ultrasound, with the statement, "I am making this election of my own free will and without coercion."

In Texas, no provision or exception exists for victims of rape or incest or in the case of a severely malformed fetus to the mandatory ultrasound requirement. Women seeking an abortion of a conception resulting from these causes are required to fulfill the informed consent criteria. Informed consent is *not* required in cases of medical emergency in which the mother's life or one of her major body functions is at risk. The physician carrying out the abortion has to certify the specific medical condition that necessitated the medical emergency.

STATE INFLUENCE AND UNDUE BURDEN

Proponents of mandatory ultrasound ask what is wrong with ensuring that a woman facing the difficult decision of aborting a fetus has access to all available information that bears on the consequences of her action and the resources available to her. After all, no one is telling her that she can or cannot proceed with the abortion. The U.S. Supreme Court stated in *Planned Parenthood of Southeast Pennsylvania vs. Casey* 505 U.S. 833, 852 (1992) that "abortion is a unique act fraught with consequences . . . for the woman must live with her decision." Opponents counter that, while full disclosure is laudable, the intent of the requirement is clearly to influence the woman's decision in the direction of not aborting. By requiring the mandatory ultrasound, opponents argue that the state assumes that a woman consenting to an abortion does not understand the nature and consequences of the procedure and therefore must be protected against herself. A woman may desire to terminate a pregnancy for multiple reasons. They include being single and without the financial resources to raise a child, rape, incest, future plans that do not involve motherhood, or the belief that she has the right number of children. While individuals may differ on whether they personally consider all of these reasons sufficient grounds for a decision to abort, they are currently legal reasons.

Oddly enough, in most states a woman's consent to put her child up for adoption is *invalid* if given before the child is born. Apparently, exposure to the infant and the birthing experience is deemed necessary for the woman to fully grasp what is at stake in giving up a child (Sanger 2008, 385).

Requiring an ultrasound before an abortion procedure poses the question of what the limits are on what the state may do to affect how certain personal choices are made and how they are implemented. Although the requirement does not appear to reach the level of a constitutional conflict, many opponents feel that the regulation places an undue burden on the woman because it has an effect or purpose other than simply to inform her consent. "[U]nnecessary health regulations that have the purpose or effect of presenting a substantial obstacle to a woman seeking an abortion impose an undue burden on the right" (*Planned Parenthood of Southeast. Pennsylvania. v. Casey*, 505 U.S. 878, 1992). The woman is coerced by law into having an ultrasound performed and then is coerced into having to refuse to view the results. Not all requirements have been judged an undue burden. A cooling off period before undergoing the procedure was not considered undue by the U.S. Supreme Court, but a requirement for spousal notification of intending to abort was rejected as just another obstacle. In other ways, mandatory ultrasound disrupts the traditional respect the law has shown for privacy, bodily integrity, and personal autonomy in decision making in reproduction, pregnancy, and family formation.

ULTRASOUND AS AN EMOTIONAL PERSUADER

The fetal ultrasound has become a cultural icon in American society that has replaced the "quickening" or first movements of a fetus felt by a pregnant woman as a sign ushering her into the sacred society of motherhood. Since the 1980s, nearly all pregnant women in the United States receive at least one ultrasound exam during the course of their pregnancy. Some go through the process multiple times during routine prenatal obstetrical care. It is so routine that specific informed consent for the procedure is not obtained, much like asking for a urine specimen. An ultrasound image now has its own cultural force. The fetus is something that can have its picture taken. It is "expected to work upon the viewer an emotional transformation, which would in turn inspire the desired behavior" (Taylor 1998).

A sonogram, however, is not like a regular photograph. It is indistinct, requiring a certain amount of training and skill to interpret the shifting, fuzzy shadows. The woman, and now often couples, are shown a gray blur on the monitor as the sonographer tells them about "their baby." They must rely on her, and sonographers are most frequently women, to tell them what they are seeing. Her tone, manner, and the vocabulary she chooses to use to describe the image are highly influential on the perceptions and emotions of the woman. Yet, in most cases, the sonographer is a technician who has no information about either the medical or personal circumstances of the patient. In a mandatory ultrasound, the sonographer is in a critical position to sway the patient's decision, yet is allowed considerable latitude on what is appropriate to say or do. Is the information being conveyed intended to help or to haunt?

Opponents of mandatory ultrasound point out that the purpose of the ultrasound is to reinforce the state's position that the fetus is not just "potential life" but is "actual life." This is despite the *lack* of consensus in the medical community that an embryo is a complete, separate, unique, and irreplaceable human being. An image, even if it has to be interpreted by a trained technician or an expert carries a deep meaning. Images evoke more of an emotional attachment than a few squiggles of a pen on chart paper, equally undecipherable as an ultrasound to the average patient. There would be less issue if "an ultrasound exam were a little more like an EKG and a little less like a visit to the hospital nursery" (Taylor 2002).

ISSUES OF PROTECTED CHOICE

Opponents of mandatory ultrasounds argue that legislating the procedure strays uncomfortably close to improperly influencing certain choices that should remain with the individual. In a liberal democracy, there are a number of decisions in which the state is held not to interfere. Examples include whether and who to marry, whether and whom to vote for, and whether and what religion to practice. The state cannot require religious education nor require nonbelievers to attend religious services to experience what they have been missing. Both the decision itself and the path taken to arrive at that decision are "protected choices."

An inexact but strikingly parallel example to mandatory ultrasound before an abortion could be encountered when renewing your driver's license (Sanger 2008, 393–394). Suppose that after filling out the forms, when you were asked to sign an organ donation card you wished to decline. Suppose additionally that before declining you were required by the state to view photographs of people on the donor list for organs, and you were informed that by checking "no" that some of those people were likely to die as a result of your decision. You also are offered the opportunity to hear recorded messages or perhaps view a short video from individuals on the list. The photographs with asterisks marked people who had died waiting for a donor. You are perfectly within your rights to decline, but showing or offering you the opportunity to view the photographs of potential victims, purely to inform your decision, is likely have an effect on your decision and how you feel about it.

CHAPTER 20

The 2009 Mammography Guidelines Controversy

Since 2002 American women have been counseled by the U.S. Preventive Services Task Force Advisory Panel to have annual or biennial mammograms starting at age forty, or earlier if there are predisposing conditions. Monthly breast self-examination was taught in an effort to catch breast cancer early. A massive education initiative carried out by physicians, educators, and organizations such as the American Cancer Society stressed the importance of early detection for the best chance of successful treatment. Their efforts were rewarded by increased public screening participation in many sectors of society as well as Medicare and expanded insurance coverage, which produced improvements in mortality due to earlier detection. Thirty-five million women have mammograms each year in the United States, at a cost of over $5 billion. Mammography screening and associated services are now big business. Demographic projections forecast breast cancer diagnosis as a growth industry. The difficulty of accurately diagnosing early breast cancer and the changing advice on mammography over time, though, has embroiled the field in continuous controversy (Finkel 2005).

On November 18, 2009, the same U.S. Preventive Services Task Force, a government-appointed but independent expert advisory panel of physicians, issued an updated set of recommendations for primary care physicians on the use of mammography in screening nonsymptomatic women for breast cancer. The new recommendations shocked women, the American Cancer Society, and other organizations concerned with breast cancer.

The Guide to Clinical Preventive Services, 2nd Edition states in Part B, "Neoplastic Diseases," Chapter 7 "Screening for Breast Cancer":

Routine screening for breast cancer every 1−2 years, with mammography alone, or mammography and annual clinical breast examination (CBE) [*breast exam by a physician*], is recommended for women aged 50−69. There is insufficient evidence to recommend for or against routine mammography or CBE for women aged 40−49 or aged 74 and older, although recommendations for high risk women aged 40−49 or aged ≥74 may be made on other grounds (see Clinical Intervention). There is insufficient evidence to recommend for or against the use of screening CBE alone or the teaching of breast self-examination.

The report, first published in the *Annals of Internal Medicine* (U.S. Preventive Services Task Force 2009), was an update of the Task Force's original recommendation (2002). Re-evaluation was based on the observed diagnostic effectiveness of current screening methods in two Panel-commissioned studies for detecting breast cancer in women. It reversed the previous recommendation of monthly breast self-examination and yearly mammograms starting at age 40 extending through age 74. It suggested instead yearly or biennial mammograms for women between the ages of 50 and 74. The response from women, physicians, and organizations such as the American Cancer Society was vehement and critical. Many people were confused and angered by the changes in the recommendations. Upsetting the dominant paradigm ingrained in women's health was viewed as a disservice to women, breast cancer sufferers, and the campaign to reduce deaths due to breast cancer. Women 40 to 49, in particular those in whom breast cancer had been detected by mammography, felt that the report meant that saving their lives, and others in a similar situation, was not considered important. There was concern that the revised recommendations would embolden the insurance industry to now deny claims for mammography expenses for the 40 to 49 age group, which accounts for almost 30 percent of mammograms, and that Medicare would refuse to cover mammograms for women over 74.

The Task Force was taken aback at the magnitude and intensity of the public response. They felt that they were simply suggesting that at age forty a woman should be consulting with her physician about whether mammography would likely be of benefit in her case, not to indicate that a mammogram should not be performed. In retrospect, the Task Force realized that the subtle language of the recommendation had not communicated the message the way they had intended. The Task Force is charged with the systematic review of preventive (diagnostic) medical services such as immunizations, counseling, screenings, and chemopreventive regimens. They periodically take into account new scientific evidence and new technologies that might be applicable.

Breast cancer detection is 1 of 169 preventive services on which recommendations are made by the Panel. The utility of these services to
deliver clinical benefit and peace of mind to the patient and his or her
physician is assessed through continued analysis of clinical trials published since earlier recommendations.

Such reviews are essential because more sensitive and refined technology and more discerning clinical trial designs are continually being
developed and applied. Not all clinical trials are equally relevant to a
given clinical situation, as each is designed to ask a particular question
about a group of subjects. For instance, a study that includes only Caucasian or Hispanic subjects may not be entirely applicable to a Black
population, and vice versa, although there may be some common elements. A mixed ethnic subject population study has to enroll a much larger
number of participants in order to draw conclusions about the entire group.
Clinical trials rarely deliver clear black and white answers, because they
deal with patient populations in which multiple factors can influence clinical outcomes and compliance can vary.

The Task Force Advisory Panel

The current Panel is composed of nine members from academic medicine departments at universities and one from private practice, representing the main primary care medical specialties—internal medicine, family
medicine, obstetrics and gynecology, and pediatrics as well as analytical
procedures. They are supported by staff at the Office of Disease Control
and Health Promotion in Washington, D.C., and by a network of preventive medicine experts and various medical specialists. Although it is
sponsored by the government, the Panel's role is purely advisory. Considerable effort is made to maintain its impartiality. Its members are not
federal government employees, and the various reports and recommendations are not official guidelines of the Public Health Service or the U.S.
Department of Health and Human Services. Panel recommendations are
published in peer-reviewed medical journals and *The Guide to Clinical
Preventive Services*. They are also provided to a variety of groups
involved with clinical preventive services such as medical organizations,
specialty societies, and government agencies.

Breast Cancer Figures

Approximately 182,000 new breast cancer cases were diagnosed in
women in 1995, and there were 46,000 deaths associated with the disease. The most common risk factors for developing breast cancer are

being female, living in North America or Northern Europe, and age. The age-adjusted mortality rate has changed little since 1930, with an estimated lifetime risk of 3.6 percent of a woman dying from breast cancer. It is the leading form of cancer death for women aged 15 to 64, and the death rate is exceeded only by that from infections and motor vehicle accidents. American women develop breast cancer at an approximately linearly increasing rate with age, with 127 per 100,000 women for ages between 40 and 44 increasing to 450 per 100,000 women aged 70 to 74. U.S. demographics suggest that the ongoing aging of the population will increase the total number of breast cancer cases significantly. These figures are averages for the general population of women and incidence can vary among ethnic groups. A family history of cancer in a first degree relative such as a parent increases breast cancer risk two- to three-fold, with the highest risk being for women under 50 whose relatives were diagnosed with breast cancer before menopause. Other conditions such as previous breast cancer, proliferative noncancerous lesions detected on biopsy, late age at first pregnancy, high socioeconomic status, or high-dose radiation exposure (*not* medical X-rays, which are considered low-dose) also increase the risk of cancer. In contrast, suggested associations of breast cancer with high fat diet, obesity, oral contraceptives, or long-term estrogen replacement therapy remain unproven.

INTERPRETATION OF THE REPORT

The Panel used statistical measures to determine that there was no significant decrease overall in the number of breast cancer deaths (i.e., no demonstrable benefit) in the 40 to 49 age group among the overall population of those screened by mammography. The word "significant" in this context refers to a statistical concept rather than the use in the common language to indicate how large or how important. It is a measure of how likely it is that, if you did the same study again on another group of subjects, you would find the same result. Statistically significant benefits were, on the other hand, seen for the 50 to 59 and 60 to 69 age groups. Again, for ages ≥ 74, statistically significant benefits of screening in reducing mortality, as for the 40 to 49 age group, could not be demonstrated.

The fact that statistically significant benefits could not be demonstrated for the 40 to 49 and ≥ 74 age groups does not mean that those groups should not be screened, because there *is* a significant cancer rate in both groups. For every 1,900 women 40 to 49 years old screened, one life is saved. For every 1,340 women 50 to 59 years old, a life is saved. This measure is used rather than the number of cancers detected, because many but not all breast cancers can be successfully treated. These numbers reflect the increase in incidence of breast cancer with increasing age. The Panel's recommendation was specifically to encourage women of all ages to consult with their physician and discuss the pros and cons of mammography screening, particularly those in the 40 to 49 or ≥74 age groups.

The Panel focused on two Panel-commissioned clinical trials designed such that they could evaluate whether any of the following practices reduced breast cancer mortality: (1) mammography, (2) mammography combined with either breast self-exam or clinical breast exam, or (3) either form of breast exam alone without mammography. Because the Panel's charge was to evaluate the medical utility of diagnostic and screening procedures, this was the only criterion applied in their analysis, as it was for other preventive services. Economic, political, and social considerations were not a part of the evaluation. Focusing on medical effectiveness alone is an attempt to arrive at the least biased judgment of the utility of a service. The recommendation is designed to be only one component in policy decisions made by governmental and other organizations. Those responsible for policy formulation are expected to make the difficult and controversial decisions to create a workable mix of financial, political, and social considerations. Since the public is viewing the recommendations from a broad perspective that is heavy on different proportions of the nontechnical considerations, it is not surprising that the narrow perspective of the Panel was controversial.

The lack of reference to economic forces in the Panel recommendations may contribute to opposition from some groups, including mammogram radiologists, who may feel the pressure of public criticism for performing ineffective tests. Mammograms are a multibillion dollar industry, not including the cost of follow-up medical procedures to validate the mammography results and rule out false positive conditions. Even if women and their physicians decide in favor of screening mammograms, many worry that insurance companies will attempt to avoid paying for those mammograms outside of the age range for which they are recommended. They also worry that Medicare might stop covering mammograms for older women. So far there is little indication that insurance companies are denying mammograms, especially if a physician justifies the procedure. Since the Panel's recommendations are neither federal government guidelines nor policy incumbent for government program or agencies, Medicare coverage should not be affected.

A particularly volatile issue that has raised a great deal of anger is the impact of not recommending screening for women without high-risk conditions in the 40 to 49 or >74 age groups. Because there are significant numbers of breast cancer cases in those age groups, it is difficult for those individuals to avoid coming to the conclusion that their lives have been devalued in some way. It is hard to remember that the Panel's recommendation does not come out *against* mammography screening. Rather, it does not find enough evidence that mammography screening increases the chance of detecting breast cancer in those age groups to recommend *for* mammography screening.

RISK VERSUS BENEFIT

What harm (risk) is there in screening younger women to save that 1 in 1,900 from a death from breast cancer—what is the risk-benefit ratio? The first concern that many people have about mammography is being exposed, year after year, to ionizing X-ray radiation, fearing that the exposure itself would induce cancer. The increased risk of cancer due to radiation exposure from modern low-dose mammography equipment is considered negligible by most physicians, although that risk is not zero. A second concern stems from the relatively poor ability of mammography to distinguish benign tumors, or a common slow growing but generally noninvasive ductal carcinoma in situ (DCIS) from highly invasive metastatic cancers, which leads to the risk of overdiagnosis. Treatment of overdiagnosed individuals exposes them to additional tests and treatments that offer no benefit and come with their own negative side effects. In addition, a large fraction of abnormalities detected by mammography turn out after additional testing not to be cancerous. The proportion of these false positives is reduced in settings with highly experienced operators and interpreters and the most up-to-date equipment. Breast self-exams and even clinical breast exams have similar or even higher false positive rates than mammography. The negative effects due to anxiety from receiving a false positive diagnosis requiring retesting and perhaps a biopsy can cause unintended but significant harm, especially if the experience causes the subject to avoid later screening as they age into the groups with higher incidence of cancer. There is also a significant financial cost associated with additional tests. Because individuals react differently to this situation, women are counseled to discuss the tradeoffs of risk for benefit of screening with their physician to come to a decision about when to begin mammography screening.

What many doctors fear most is that women seeing controversy and confusing or conflicting recommendations will conclude that mammography screening simply does not work to detect cancers and stop participating in screening altogether. This, all parties, including the Panel, agree would be an unfortunate reaction and would result in an increase in breast cancer mortality due to the cancers going undetected by any method.

BETTER DIAGNOSTICS, BETTER DIAGNOSIS

One of the consequences of the 2009 recommendations controversy is that it has stimulated discussion about finding better ways to detect true breast malignancies more specifically and to reduce false positives and thus unnecessary and possibly harmful treatment. Other imaging technologies are being brought to bear on the detection problem including magnetic resonance imaging, ultrasound, and thermography. Another method using SPECT or PET imaging of a radiolabeled chemical reagent that specifically recognizes cancerous cells may have the greatest promise for specificity, although it would require exposure to ionizing radiation and would be relatively expensive. Suitable specific ligands also need to be developed. These methods are currently insufficiently advanced to challenge the gold standard, mammography, as a screening method.

Nonimaging methods, such as a blood test for the detection of breast cancer, are also potentially of screening value. Outside of a test for estrogen-responsive tumors, BCR, which will determine whether an identified tumor will respond to hormone antagonist drug treatment, there is a dearth of currently well-accepted breast cancer screening diagnostic agents. Part of the difficulty is that early detection requires high sensitivity and the ability to detect just a few cells. Imaging is well-suited for detecting localized masses of tumor cells.

The Institute of Medicine Committee of the U.S. National Academy of Sciences has identified characteristics for an "ideal" screening tool, including a low risk of harm, high specificity, noninvasive, cost-effective, and ability to distinguish slow-growing, nonprogressing lesions from those that are cancerous and life-threatening. No such tools exist at present.

PART III

References and Resources

Annotated Primary Source Documents

"THE NEW MARVEL IN PHOTOGRAPHY"

The following article by H. J. W. Dam appeared in the April 1896 issue of McClure's Magazine, *only months after the initial discovery of X-rays in November 1895. The article vividly conveys not only the swiftness with which the discovery revolutionized medicine, but also the public's amazement at being able to see inside the intact human body for the first time. While Dam clearly sees this new discovery as "epoch-making," he also hints at the alarm caused by the technology with its ability to "see through everything from a purse or a pocket to the walls of a room or a house," raising entirely new privacy issues. The article is also entertaining for Dam's colorful first-hand descriptions of Wilhelm Roentgen and for such overconfident assertions by contemporary researchers as "all the organs of the human body can, and will, shortly, be photographed."*

"The New Marvel in Photography: A Visit to Professor Röntgen at His Laboratory in Würtzburg—His Own Account of His Great Discovery—Interesting Experiments with the Cathode Rays—Practical Uses of the New Photography"

By H. J. W. Dam

In all the history of scientific discovery there has never been, perhaps, so general, rapid, and dramatic an effect wrought on the scientific centres of Europe as has followed, in the past four weeks, upon an announcement made to the Würzburg Physico-Medical Society, at their December meeting, by Professor William Konrad Röntgen, professor of physics at the Royal University of Würzburg. The first news which reached London was by telegraph from Vienna to the effect that a

Professor Röntgen, until then the possessor of only a local fame in the town mentioned, had discovered a new kind of light, which penetrated and photographed through everything. This news was received with a mild interest, some amusement, and much incredulity; and a week passed. Then, by mail and telegraph, came daily clear indications of the stir which the discovery was making in all the great line of universities between Vienna and Berlin. Then Röntgen's own report arrived, so cool, so business-like, and so truly scientific in character, that it left no doubt either of the truth or of the great importance of the preceding reports. To-day, four weeks after the announcement, Röntgen's name is apparently in every scientific publication issued this week in Europe; and accounts of his experiments, of the experiments of others following his method, and of theories as to the strange new force which he has been the first to observe, fill pages of every scientific journal that comes to hand. And before the necessary time elapses for this article to attain publication in America, it is in all ways probable that the laboratories and lecture-rooms of the United States will also be giving full evidence of this contagious arousal of interest over a discovery so strange that its importance cannot yet be measured, its utility be even prophesied, or its ultimate effect upon long-established scientific beliefs be even vaguely foretold.

The Röntgen rays are certain invisible rays resembling, in many respects, rays of light, which are set free when a high pressure electric current is discharged through a vacuum tube. A vacuum tube is a glass tube from which all the air, down to one-millionth of an atmosphere, has been exhausted after the insertion of a platinum wire in either end of the tube for connection with the two poles of a battery or induction coil. When the discharge is sent through the tube, there proceeds from the anode—that is, the wire which is connected with the positive pole of the battery—certain bands of light, varying in color with the color of the glass. But these are insignificant in comparison with the brilliant glow which shoots from the cathode, or negative wire. This glow excites brilliant phosphorescence in glass and many substances, and these "cathode rays," as they are called, were observed and studied by Hertz; and more deeply by his assistant, Professor Lenard, Lenard having, in 1894, reported that the cathode rays would penetrate thin films of aluminium, wood, and other substances and produce photographic results beyond. It was left, however, for Professor Röntgen to discover that during the discharge another kind of rays are set free, which differ greatly from those described by Lenard as cathode rays. The most marked difference between the two is the fact that Röntgen rays are not deflected by a magnet, indicating a very essential difference, while their range and penetrative power are incomparably greater. In fact, all those qualities which have lent a sensational character to the discovery of Röntgen's rays were mainly absent from these of Lenard, to the end that, although Röntgen has not been working in an entirely new field, he has by common accord been freely granted all the honors of a great discovery.

Exactly what kind of a force Professor Röntgen has discovered he does not know. As will be seen below, he declines to call it a new kind of light, or a new form of electricity. He has given it the name of the X rays. Others speak of it as the Röntgen rays. Thus far its results only, and not its essence, are known. In the terminology of science it is generally called "a new mode of motion," or, in other words, a new force. As to whether it is or not actually a force new to science, or one of the known forces masquerading under strange conditions, weighty authorities are already arguing. More than one eminent scientist has already affected to see in it a key to the great mystery of the law of gravity. All who have expressed themselves in print have admitted, with more or less frankness, that, in view of Röntgen's discovery, science must forth-with revise, possibly to a revolutionary degree, the long accepted theories concerning the phenomena of light and sound. That the X rays, in their mode of action, combine a strange resemblance to both sound and light vibrations, and are destined to materially affect, if they do not greatly alter, our views of both phenomena, is already certain; and beyond this is the opening into a new and unknown field of physical knowledge, concerning which speculation is already eager, and experimental investigation already in hand, in London, Paris, Berlin, and, perhaps, to a greater or less extent, in every well-equipped physical laboratory in Europe.

This is the present scientific aspect of the discovery. But, unlike most epoch-making results from laboratories, this discovery is one which, to a very unusual degree, is within the grasp of the popular and non-technical imagination. Among the other kinds of matter which these rays penetrate with ease is the human flesh. That a new photography has suddenly arisen which can photograph the bones, and, before long, the organs of the human body; that a light has been found which can penetrate, so as to make a photographic record, through everything from a purse or a pocket to the walls of a room or a house, is news which cannot fail to startle everybody. That the eye of the physician or surgeon, long baffled by the skin, and vainly seeking to penetrate the unfortunate darkness of the human body, is now to be supplemented by a camera, making all the parts of the human body as visible, in a way, as the exterior, appears certainly to be a greater blessing to humanity than even the Listerian antiseptic system of surgery; and its benefits must inevitably be greater than those conferred by Lister, great as the latter have been. Already, in the few weeks since Röntgen's announcement, the results of surgical operations under the new system are growing voluminous. In Berlin, not only new bone fractures are being immediately photographed, but joined fractures, as well, in order to examine the results of recent surgical work. In Vienna, imbedded bullets are being photographed, instead of being probed for, and extracted with comparative ease. In London, a wounded sailor, completely paralyzed, whose injury was a mystery, has been saved by the photographing of an object imbedded in the spine, which, upon extraction, proved to be a small knife-blade. Operations for malformations, hitherto obscure, but now clearly revealed by the new photography, are already becoming common, and are being reported from all directions. Professor Czermark of Graz has photographed the living skull, denuded of flesh and hair, and has begun the adaptation of the new photography to brain study. The relation of the new rays to thought rays is being eagerly discussed in what may be called the non-exact circles and journals; and all that numerous group of inquirers into the occult, the believers in clairvoyance, spiritualism, telepathy, and kindred orders of alleged phenomena, are confident of finding in the new force long-sought facts in proof of their claims. Professor Neusser in Vienna has photographed gall-stones in the liver of one patient (the stone showing snow-white in the negative), and a stone in the bladder of another patient. His results so far induce him to announce that all the organs of the human body can, and will, shortly, be photographed. Lannelougue of Paris has exhibited to the Academy of Science photographs of bones showing inherited tuberculosis which had not otherwise revealed itself. Berlin has already formed a society of forty for the immediate prosecution of researches into both the character of the new force and its physiological possibilities. In the next few weeks these strange announcements will be trebled or quadrupled, giving the best evidence from all quarters of the great future that awaits the Röntgen rays, and the startling impetus to the universal search for knowledge that has come at the close of the nineteenth century from the modest little laboratory in the Pleicher Ring at Würzburg.

On instruction by cable from the editor of this magazine, on the first announcement of the discovery, I set out for Würzburg to see the discoverer and his laboratory. I found a neat and thriving Bavarian city of forty-five thousand inhabitants, which, for some ten centuries, has made no salient claim upon the admiration of the world, except for the elaborateness of its mediæval castle and the excellence of its local beer. Its streets were adorned with large numbers of students, all wearing either scarlet, green, or blue caps, and an extremely serious expression, suggesting much intensity either in the contemplation of Röntgen rays or of the beer aforesaid. All knew the residence of Professor Röntgen (pronunciation: "Renken"), and directed me to the "Pleicher Ring." The various buildings of the university are scattered in different parts of Würzburg, the majority being in the Pleicher Ring, which is a fine avenue, with a park along one side of it, in the centre of the town. The Physical Institute, Professor Röntgen's particular domain, is a modest building of two stories and basement, the upper story constituting his private residence, and the remainder of the building being given over to lecture rooms, laboratories, and their attendant offices. At the door I was met by an old serving-man of the idolatrous order, whose pain was apparent when I asked for "Professor" Röntgen, and he gently corrected me with "Herr Doctor Röntgen." As it was evident, however, that we referred to the same person, he conducted me along a wide, bare hall, running the length of the building, with blackboards and charts on the walls. At the end he showed me into a small room on the right. This contained a large table desk, and a small table by the window, covered with photographs, while the walls held rows of shelves laden with laboratory and other records. An open door led into a somewhat larger room, perhaps twenty feet by fifteen, and I found myself gazing into a laboratory which was the scene of the discovery—a laboratory which, though in all ways modest, is destined to be enduringly historical.

There was a wide table shelf running along the farther side, in front of the two windows, which were high, and gave plenty of light. In the centre was a stove; on the left, a small cabinet, whose shelves held the small objects which the professor had been using. There was a table in the left-hand corner; and another small table—the one on which living bones were first photographed—was near the stove, and a Rhumkorff coil was on the right. The lesson of the laboratory was eloquent. Compared, for instance, with the elaborate, expensive, and complete apparatus of, say, the University of London, or of any of the great American universities, it was bare and unassuming to a degree. It mutely said that in the great march of science it is the genius of man, and not the perfection of appliances, that breaks new ground in the great territory of the unknown. It also caused one to wonder at and endeavor to imagine the great things which are to be done through elaborate appliances with the Röntgen rays—a field in which the United States, with its foremost genius in invention, will very possibly, if not probably, take the lead—when the discoverer himself had done so much with so little. Already, in a few weeks, a skilled London operator, Mr. A. A. C. Swinton, has reduced the necessary time of exposure for Röntgen photographs from fifteen minutes to four. He used, however, a Tesla oil coil, discharged by twelve half-gallon Leyden jars, with an alternating current of twenty thousand volts' pressure. Here were no oil coils, Leyden jars, or specially elaborate and expensive machines. There were only a Rhumkorff coil and Crookes (vacuum) tube and the man himself.

Professor Röntgen entered hurriedly, something like an amiable gust of wind. He is a tall, slender, and loose-limbed man, whose whole appearance bespeaks enthusiasm and energy. He wore a dark blue sack suit, and his long, dark hair stood straight up from his forehead, as if he were permanently electrified by his own enthusiasm. His voice is full and deep, he speaks rapidly, and, altogether, he seems clearly a man who, once upon the track of a mystery which appealed to him, would pursue it with unremitting vigor. His eyes are kind, quick, and penetrating; and there is no doubt that he much prefers gazing at a Crookes tube to beholding a visitor, visitors at present robbing him of much valued time. The meeting was by appointment, however, and his greeting was cordial and hearty. In addition to his own language he speaks French well and English scientifically, which is different from speaking it popularly. These three tongues being more or less within the equipment of his visitor, the conversation proceeded on an international or polyglot basis, so to speak, varying at necessity's demand.

It transpired, in the course of inquiry, that the professor is a married man and fifty years of age, though his eyes have the enthusiasm of twenty-five. He was born near Zurich, and educated there, and completed his studies and took his degree at Utrecht. He has been at Würzburg about seven years, and had made no discoveries which he considered of great importance prior to the one under consideration. These details were given under good-natured protest, he failing to understand why his personality should interest the public. He declined to admire himself or his results in any degree, and laughed at the idea of being famous. The professor is too deeply interested in science to waste any time in thinking about himself. His emperor had fêted, flattered, and decorated him, and he was loyally grateful. It was evident, however, that fame and applause had small attractions for him, compared to the mysteries still hidden in the vacuum tubes of the other room.

"Now, then," said he, smiling, and with some impatience, when the pre-liminary questions at which he chafed were over, "you have come to see the invisible rays."

"Is the invisible visible?"

"Not to the eye; but its results are. Come in here."

He led the way to the other square room mentioned, and indicated the induction coil with which his researches were made, an ordinary Rhumkorff coil, with a spark of from four to six inches, charged by a current of twenty **amperes**. Two wires led from the coil, through an open door, into a smaller room on the right. In this room was a small table carrying a Crookes tube connected with the coil. The most striking object in the room, however, was a huge and mysterious tin box about seven feet high and four feet square. It stood on end, like a huge packing-case, its side being perhaps five inches from the Crookes tube.

The professor explained the mystery of the tin box, to the effect that it was a device of his own for obtaining a portable dark-room. When he began his investigations he used the whole room, as was shown by the heavy blinds and curtains so arranged as to exclude the entrance of all interfering light from the windows. In the side of the tin box, at the point immediately against the tube, was a circular sheet of aluminium one millimetre in thickness, and perhaps eighteen inches in diameter, soldered to the surrounding tin. To study his rays the professor had only to turn on the current, enter the box, close the door, and in perfect darkness inspect only such light or light effects as he had a right to consider his own, hiding his light, in fact, not under the Biblical bushel, but in a more commodious box.

"Step inside," said he, opening the door, which was on the side of the box far-thest from the tube. I immediately did so, not altogether certain whether my skele-ton was to be photographed for general inspection, or my secret thoughts held up to light on a glass plate. "You will find a sheet of barium paper on the shelf," he added, and then went away to the coil. The door was closed, and the interior of the box became black darkness. The first thing I found was a wooden stool, on which I resolved to sit. Then I found the shelf on the side next the tube, and then the sheet of paper prepared with barium platino-cyanide. I was thus being shown the first phenomenon which attracted the discoverer's attention and led to the discovery, namely, the passage of rays, themselves wholly invisible, whose presence was only indicated by the effect they produced on a piece of sensitized photographic paper.

A moment later, the black darkness was penetrated by the rapid snapping sound of the high-pressure current in action, and I knew that the tube outside was glowing. I held the sheet vertically on the shelf, perhaps four inches from the plate. There was no change, however, and nothing was visible.

"Do you see anything?" he called.

"No."

"The tension is not high enough;" and he proceeded to increase the pressure by operating an apparatus of mercury in long vertical tubes acted upon automatically by a weight lever which stood near the coil. In a few moments the sound of the discharge again began, and then I made my first acquaintance with the Röntgen rays.

The moment the current passed, the paper began to glow. A yellowish-green light spread all over its surface in clouds, waves, and flashes. The yellow-green luminescence, all the stranger and stronger in the darkness, trembled, wavered, and floated over the paper, in rhythm with the snapping of the discharge. Through the metal plate, the paper, myself, and the tin box, the invisible rays were flying, with an effect strange, interesting, and uncanny. The metal plate seemed to offer no appreciable resistance to the flying force, and the light was as rich and full as if nothing lay between the paper and the tube.

"Put the book up," said the professor.

I felt upon the shelf, in the darkness, a heavy book, two inches in thickness, and placed this against the plate. It made no difference. The rays flew through the metal and the book as if neither had been there, and the waves of light, rolling cloud-like over the paper, showed no change in brightness. It was a clear, material illustration of the ease with which paper and wood are penetrated. And then I laid book and paper down, and put my eyes against the rays. All was blackness, and I neither saw nor felt anything. The discharge was in full force, and the rays were flying through my head, and, for all I knew, through the side of the box behind me. But they were invisible and impalpable. They gave no sensation whatever. Whatever the mysterious rays may be, they are not to be seen, and are to be judged only by their works.

I was loath to leave this historical tin box, but time pressed. I thanked the professor, who was happy in the reality of his discovery and the music of his sparks. Then I said: "Where did you first photograph living bones?"

"Here," he said, leading the way into the room where the coil stood. He pointed to a table on which was another—the latter a small short-legged wooden one with more the shape and size of a wooden seat. It was two feet square and painted coal black. I viewed it with interest. I would have bought it, for the little table on which light was first sent through the human body will some day be a great historical curiosity; but it was "nicht zu verkaufen." A photograph of it would have been a consolation, but for several reasons one was not to be had at present. However, the historical table was there, and was duly inspected.

"How did you take the first hand photograph?" I asked.

The professor went over to a shelf by the window, where lay a number of prepared glass plates, closely wrapped in black paper. He put a Crookes tube underneath the table, a few inches from the under side of its top. Then he laid his hand flat on the top of the table, and placed the glass plate loosely on his hand.

"You ought to have your portrait painted in that attitude," I suggested.

"No, that is nonsense," said he, smiling.

"Or be photographed." This suggestion was made with a deeply hidden purpose.

The rays from the Röntgen eyes instantly penetrated the deeply hidden purpose. "Oh, no," said he; "I can't let you make pictures of me. I am too busy." Clearly the professor was entirely too modest to gratify the wishes of the curious world.

"Now, Professor," said I, "will you tell me the history of the discovery?"

"There is no history," he said. "I have been for a long time interested in the problem of the cathode rays from a vacuum tube as studied by Hertz and Lenard. I had followed theirs and other researches with great interest, and determined, as soon as I had the time, to make some researches of my own. This time I found at the close of last October. I had been at work for some days when I discovered something new."

"What was the date?"

"The eighth of November."

"And what was the discovery?"

"I was working with a Crookes tube covered by a shield of black cardboard. A piece of barium platino-cyanide paper lay on the bench there. I had been passing a current through the tube, and I noticed a peculiar black line across the paper."

"What of that?"

"The effect was one which could only be produced, in ordinary parlance, by the passage of light. No light could come from the tube, because the shield which covered it was impervious to any light known, even that of the electric arc."

"And what did you think?"

"I did not think; I investigated. I assumed that the effect must have come from the tube, since its character indicated that it could come from nowhere else. I tested it. In a few minutes there was no doubt about it. Rays were coming from the tube which had a luminescent effect upon the paper. I tried it successfully at greater and greater distances, even at two metres. It seemed at first a new kind of invisible light. It was clearly something new, something unrecorded."

"Is it light?"

"No."

"Is it electricity?"

"Not in any known form."

"What is it?"

"I don't know."

And the discoverer of the X rays thus stated as calmly his ignorance of their essence as has everybody else who has written on the phenomena thus far.

"Having discovered the existence of a new kind of rays, I of course began to investigate what they would do." He took up a series of cabinet-sized photographs. "It soon appeared from tests that the rays had penetrative power to a degree hitherto unknown. They penetrated paper, wood, and cloth with ease; and the thickness of the substance made no perceptible difference, within reasonable limits." He showed photographs of a box of laboratory weights of platinum, aluminium, and brass, they and the brass hinges all having been photographed from a closed box, without any indication of the box. Also a photograph of a coil of fine wire, wound on a wooden spool, the wire having been photographed, and the wood omitted. "The rays," he continued, "passed through all the metals tested, with a facility varying, roughly speaking, with the density of the metal. These phenomena I have discussed carefully in my report to the Würzburg society, and you will find all the technical results therein stated." He showed a photograph of a small sheet of zinc. This was composed of smaller plates soldered laterally with solders of different metallic proportions. The differing lines of shadow, caused by the difference in the solders, were visible evidence that a new means of detecting flaws and chemical variations in metals had been found. A photograph of a compass showed the needle and dial taken through the closed brass cover. The markings of the dial were in red metallic paint, and thus interfered with the rays, and were reproduced. "Since the rays had this great penetrative power, it seemed natural that they should penetrate flesh, and so it proved in photographing the hand, as I showed you."

A detailed discussion of the characteristics of his rays the professor considered unprofitable and unnecessary. He believes, though, that these mysterious radiations are not light, because their behavior is essentially different from that of light rays, even those light rays which are themselves invisible. The Röntgen rays cannot be reflected by reflecting surfaces, concentrated by lenses, or refracted or diffracted. They produce photographic action on a sensitive film, but their action is weak as yet, and herein lies the first important field of their development. The professor's exposures were comparatively long—an average of fifteen minutes in easily penetrable media, and half an hour or more in photographing the bones of the hand. Concerning vacuum tubes, he said that he preferred the Hittorf, because it had the most perfect vacuum, the highest degree of air exhaustion being the consummation most desirable. In answer to a question, "What of the future?" he said:

"I am not a prophet, and I am opposed to prophesying. I am pursuing my investigations, and as fast as my results are verified I shall make them public."

"Do you think the rays can be so modified as to photograph the organs of the human body?"

In answer he took up the photograph of the box of weights. "Here are already modifications," he said, indicating the various degrees of shadow produced by the aluminium, platinum, and brass weights, the brass hinges, and even the metallic stamped lettering on the cover of the box, which was faintly perceptible.

"But Professor Neusser has already announced that the photographing of the various organs is possible."

"We shall see what we shall see," he said. We have the start now; the developments will follow in time."

"You know the apparatus for introducing the electric light into the stomach?"

"Yes."

"Do you think that this electric light will become a vacuum tube for photographing, from the stomach, any part of the abdomen or thorax?"

The idea of swallowing a Crookes tube, and sending a high frequency current down into one's stomach, seemed to him exceedingly funny. "When I have done it, I will tell you," he said, smiling, resolute in abiding by results.

"There is much to do, and I am busy, very busy," he said in conclusion. He extended his hand in farewell, his eyes already wandering toward his work in the inside room. And his visitor promptly left him; the words, "I am busy," said in all sincerity, seeming to describe in a single phrase the essence of his character and the watchword of a very unusual man.

Returning by way of Berlin, I called upon Herr Spies of the Urania, whose photographs after the Röntgen method were the first made public, and have been the best seen thus far. The Urania is a peculiar institution, and one which it seems might be profitably duplicated in other countries. It is a scientific theatre. By means of the lantern and an admirable equipment of scientific appliances, all new discoveries, as well as ordinary interesting and picturesque phenomena, when new discoveries are lacking, are described and illustrated daily to the public, who pay for seats as in an ordinary theatre, and keep the Urania profitably filled all the year round. Professor Spies is a young man of great mental alertness and mechanical resource. It is the photograph of a hand, his wife's hand, which illustrates, perhaps better than any other illustration in this article, the clear delineation of the bones which can be obtained by the Röntgen rays. In speaking of the discovery he said:

"I applied it, as soon as the penetration of flesh was apparent, to the photograph of a man's hand. Something in it had pained him for years, and the photograph at once exhibited a small foreign object, as you can see;" and he exhibited a copy of the photograph in question. "The speck there is a small piece of glass, which was immediately extracted, and which, in all probability, would have otherwise remained in the man's hand to the end of his days." All of which indicates that the needle which has pursued its travels in so many persons, through so many years, will be suppressed by the camera.

"My next object is to photograph the bones of the entire leg," continued Herr Spies. "I anticipate no difficulty, though it requires some thought in manipulation."

It will be seen that the Röntgen rays and their marvellous practical possibilities are still in their infancy. The first successful modification of the action of the rays so that the varying densities of bodily organs will enable them to be photographed, will bring all such morbid growths as tumors and cancers into the photographic field, to say nothing of vital organs which may be abnormally developed or degenerate. How much this means to medical and surgical practice it requires little imagination to conceive. Diagnosis, long a painfully uncertain science, has received an unexpected and wonderful assistant; and how greatly the world will benefit thereby, how much pain will be saved, and how many lives saved, the future can only determine. In science a new door has been opened where none was known to exist, and a side-light on phenomena has appeared, of which the results may prove as penetrating and astonishing as the Röntgen rays themselves. The most agreeable feature of the discovery is the opportunity it gives for other hands to help; and the work of these hands will add many new words to the dictionaries, many new facts to science, and, in the years long ahead of us, fill many more volumes than there are paragraphs in this brief and imperfect account.

"THE RÖNTGEN RAYS IN AMERICA"

The following article by Cleveland Moffett, also appearing in the April 1896 issue of McClure's Magazine, *paints a dramatic picture of the flurry of scientific research in the United States in the months immediately following the discovery of X-rays.*

"The Röntgen Rays in America"

By Cleveland Moffett

At the top of the great Sloane laboratory of Yale University, in an experimenting room lined with curious apparatus, I found Professor Arthur W. Wright experimenting with the wonderful Röntgen rays. Professor Wright, a small, low-voiced man, of modest manner, has achieved, in his experiments in photographing through solid substances, some of the most interesting and remarkable results thus far attained in this country. His success is, no doubt, largely due to the fact that for years he had been experimenting constantly with vacuum tubes similar to the Crookes tubes used in producing the cathode rays.

When I arrived, Professor Wright was at work with a Crookes tube, nearly spherical in shape, and about five inches in diameter—the one with which he has taken all his shadow pictures. His best results have been obtained with long exposures—an hour or an hour and a half—and he regards it as of the first importance that the objects through which the Röntgen rays are to be projected be placed as near as possible to the sensitized plate.

It is from a failure to observe this precaution that so many of the shadow pictures show blurred outlines. It is with these pictures as with a shadow of the hand thrown on the wall—the nearer the hand is to the wall, the more distinct becomes the shadow; and this consideration makes Professor Wright doubt whether it will be possible, with the present facilities, to get clearly cut shadow images of very thick objects, or in cases where the pictures are taken through a thick board or other obstacle. The Röntgen rays will doubtless traverse the board, and shadows will be formed upon the plate, but there will be an uncertainty or dimness of outline that will render the results unsatisfactory. It is for this reason that Professor Wright has taken most of his shadow pictures through only the thickness of ebonite in his plate-holder. A most successful shadow picture taken by Professor Wright in this way, shows five objects laid side by side on a large plate—a saw, a case of pocket tools in their cover, a pocket lense opened out as for use, a pair of eye-glasses inside their leather case, and an awl. As will be seen from the accompanying reproduction of this picture, all the objects are photographed with remarkable distinctness, the leather case of the eye-glasses being almost transparent, the wood of the handles of the awl and saw being a little less so, while the glass in the eye-glasses is less transparent than either. In the case of the awl and the saw, the iron stem of the tool shows plainly inside the wooden handle. This photograph is similar to a dozen that have been taken by Professor Wright with equal success. The exposure here was fifty-five minutes.

A more remarkable picture is one taken in the same way, but with a somewhat longer exposure—of a rabbit laid upon the ebonite plate, and so successfully pierced with the Röntgen rays that not only the bones of the body show plainly, but also the six grains of shot with which the animal was killed. The bones of the fore legs show with beautiful distinctness inside the shadowy flesh, while a closer inspection makes visible the ribs, the cartilages of the ear, and a lighter region in the centre of the body, which marks the location of the heart.

Like most experimenters, Professor Wright has taken numerous shadow pictures of the human hand, showing the bones within, and he has made a great number of experiments in photographing various metals and different varieties of quartz and glass, with a view to studying characteristic differences in the shadows produced. A photograph of the latter sort is reproduced on page 401. Aluminium shows a remarkable degree of transparency to the Röntgen rays; so much so that Professor Wright was able to photograph a medal of this metal, showing in the same picture the designs and lettering on both sides of the medal, presented simultaneously in superimposed images. The denser metals, however, give in the main black shadows, which offer little opportunity of distinguishing between them.

As to the nature of the Röntgen rays, Professor Wright is inclined to regard them as a mode of motion through the ether, in longitudinal stresses; and he thinks that, while they are in many ways similar to the rays discovered by Lenard a year or so ago, they still present important characteristics of their own. It may be, he thinks, that the Röntgen rays are the ordinary cathode rays produced in a Crookes tube, filtered, if one may so express it, of the metallic particles carried in their electrical stream from the metal terminal, on passing through the glass. It is well known that the metal terminals of a Crookes tube are steadily worn away while the current is passing; so much so that sometimes portions of the interior of the tube become coated with a metallic deposit almost mirror-like.

As to the future, Professor Wright feels convinced that important results will be achieved in surgery and medicine by the use of these new rays, while in physical science they point to an entirely new field of investigation. The most necessary thing now is to find some means of producing streams of Röntgen rays of greater volume and intensity, so as to make possible greater penetration and distinctness in the images. Thus far only small Crookes tubes have been used, and much is to be expected when larger ones become available; but there is great difficulty in the manufacture of them. It might be possible, Professor Wright thinks, to get good results by using, instead of the Crookes tube, a large sphere of aluminium, which is more transparent to the new rays than glass and possesses considerable strength. It is a delicate question, however, whether the increased thickness of metal necessary to resist the air pressure upon a vacuum would not offset the advantage gained from the greater size. Moreover, it is a matter for experiment still to determine, what kind of an electric current would be necessary to excite such a larger tube with the best results.

Among the most important experiments in shadow photography made thus far in America are those of Dr. William J. Morton of New York, who was the first in this country to use the disruptive discharges of static electricity in connection with the Röntgen discovery, and to demonstrate that shadow pictures may be successfully taken without the use of Crookes tubes. It was the well-known photographic properties of ordinary lightning that made Dr. Morton suspect that cathode rays are produced freely in the air when there is an electric discharge from the heavens. Reasoning thus, he resolved to search for cathode rays in the ten-inch lightning flash he was able to produce between the poles of his immense Holtz machine, probably the largest in this country.

On January 30th he suspended a glass plate, with a circular window in the middle, between the two poles. Cemented to this plate of glass was one of hard rubber, about equal in size, which of course covered the window in the glass. Back of the rubber plate was suspended a photographic plate in the plate-holder, and outside of this, between it and the rubber surface, were ten letters cut from thin copper. Dr. Morton proposed to see if he could not prove the existence of cathode rays between the poles by causing them to picture in shadow, upon the sensitized plate, the letters thus exposed.

In order to do this it was necessary to separate the ordinary electric sparks from the invisible cathode rays which, as Dr. Morton believed, accompanied them. It was to accomplish this that he used the double plates of glass and hard rubber placed, as already described, between the two poles; for while the ordinary electric spark would not traverse the rubber, any cathode rays that might be present would do so with great ease, the circular window in the glass plate allowing them passage there.

The current being turned on, it was found that the powerful electric sparks visible to the eye, unable to follow a straight course on account of the intervening rubber plate, jumped around the two plates in jagged, lightning-like lines, and thus reached the other pole of the machine. But it was noticed that at the same time a faint spray of purplish light was streaming straight through the rubber between the two holes, as if its passage was not interfered with by the rubber plate. It was in company with this stream of violet rays, known as the brush discharge, that the doctor conceived the invisible Röntgen rays to be projected at each spark discharge around the plate; and presently, when the photographic plate was developed, it was found that his conception was based on fact. For there, dim in outline, but unmistakable, were shadow pictures of the ten letters which stand as historic, since they were probably the first shadow pictures in the world taken without any bulb or vacuum tube whatever. These shadow pictures Dr. Morton carefully distinguished from the ordinary blackening effects on the film produced by electrified objects.

Pursuing his experiments with static electricity, Dr. Morton soon found that better results could be obtained by the use of Leyden jars influenced by the Holtz machine, and discharging into a vacuum bulb, as shown in the illustration on this page. This arrangement of the apparatus has the advantage of making it much easier to regulate the electric supply and to modify its intensity, and Dr. Morton finds that in this way large vacuum tubes, perhaps twenty inches in diameter, may be excited to the point of doing practical work without danger of breaking the glass walls. But certain precautions are necessary. When he uses tin-foil electrodes on the outside of the bulb, he protects the tin-foil edges, and, what is more essential, uses extremely small Leyden jars and a short spark gap between the poles of the discharging rods. The philosophy of this is, that the smaller the jars, the greater their number of oscillations per second (easily fifteen million, according to Dr. Lodge's computations), the shorter the wave length, and, therefore, the greater the intensity of effects.

The next step was to bring more energy into play, still using Leyden jars; and for this purpose Dr. Morton placed within the circuit between the jars a Tesla oscillating coil. He was thus able to use in his shadow pictures the most powerful sparks the machine was capable of producing (twelve inches), sending the Leyden-jar discharge through the primary of the coil, and employing for the excitation of the vacuum tube the "step up" current of the secondary coil with a potential incalculably increased.

While Dr. Morton has in some of his experiments excited his Leyden jars from an induction coil, he thinks the best promise lies in the use of powerful Holtz machines; and he now uses no Leyden jars or converters, thus greatly adding to the simplicity of operations.

In regard to the bulb, Dr. Morton has tested various kinds of vacuum tubes, the ordinary Crookes tubes, the Geissler tubes, and has obtained excellent results from the use of a special vacuum lamp adapted by himself to the purpose. One of his ingenious expedients was to turn to use an ordinary radiometer of large bulb, and, having fitted this with tin-foil electrodes, he found that he was able to get strongly marked shadow pictures. This application of the Röntgen principle will commend itself to many students who, being unable to provide themselves with the rare and expensive Crookes tubes, may buy a radiometer which will serve their purpose excellently in any laboratory supply store, the cost being only a few dollars, while the application of the tin foil electrodes is perfectly simple.

In the-well equipped Jackson laboratory at Trinity College, Hartford, I found Dr. W. L. Robb, the professor of physics, surrounded by enthusiastic students, who were assisting him in some experiments with the new rays. Dr. Robb is the better qualified for this work from the fact that he pursued his electrical studies at the Würzburg University, in the very laboratory where Professor Röntgen made his great discovery. The picture reproduced herewith, showing a human foot inside the shoe, was taken by Dr. Robb. The Crookes tubes used in this and in most of Dr. Robb's experiments are considerably larger than any I have seen elsewhere, being pear-shaped, about eight inches long, and four inches wide at the widest part. It is, perhaps, to the excellence of this tube that Dr. Robb owes part of his success. At any rate, in the foot picture the bones are outlined through shoe and stocking, while every nail in the sole of the shoe shows plainly, although the rays came from above, striking the top of the foot first, the sole resting upon the plate-holder. In other of Dr. Robb's pictures equally fine results were obtained; notably in one of a fish, reproduced herewith, and showing the bony structure of the body; one of a razor, where the lighter shadow proves that the hollow ground portion is almost as thin as the edge; and one of a man's hand, taken for use in a lawsuit, to prove that the bones of the thumb, which had been crushed and broken in an accident, had been improperly set by the attending physician.

Dr. Robb has made a series of novel and important experiments with tubes from which the air has been exhausted in varying degrees, and has concluded from these that it is impossible to produce the Röntgen phenomena unless there is present in the tube an almost perfect vacuum. Through a tube half exhausted, on connecting it with an induction coil, he obtained merely the ordinary series of sparks; in a tube three-quarters exhausted, he obtained a reddish glow from end to end, a torpedo-shaped stream of fire; through a tube exhausted to a fairly high degree—what the electric companies would call "not bad"—he obtained a beautiful streaked effect of bluish striæ in transverse layers. Finally, in a tube exhausted as highly as possible, he obtained a faint fluorescent glow, like that produced in a Crookes tube. This fluorescence of the glass, according to Dr. Robb, invariably accompanies the discharge of Röntgen rays, and it is likely that these rays are produced more abundantly as the fluorescence increases. Just how perfect a vacuum is needed to give the best results remains a matter of conjecture. It is possible, of course, as Tesla believes, that with an absolutely perfect vacuum no results whatever would be obtained.

Dr. Robb has discovered that in order to get the best results with shadow pictures it is necessary to use special developers for the plates, and a different process in the dark-room from the one known to ordinary photographers. In a general way, it is necessary to use solutions designed to affect the ultra-violet rays, and not the visible rays of the spectrum. Having succeeded, after much experiment, in thus modifying his developing process to meet the needs of the case, Dr. Robb finds that he makes a great gain in time of exposure, fifteen minutes being sufficient for the average shadow picture taken through a layer of wood or leather, and half an hour representing an extreme case. In some shadow pictures, as, for instance, in taking a lead-pencil, it is a great mistake to give an exposure exceeding two or three minutes; for the wood is so transparent that with a long exposure it does not show at all, and the effect of the picture is spoiled. Indeed, Dr. Robb finds that there is a constant tendency to shorten the time of exposure, and with good results. For instance, one of the best shadow pictures he had taken was of a box of instruments covered by two thicknesses of leather, two thicknesses of velvet, and two thicknesses of wood; and yet the time of exposure, owing to an accident to the coil, was only five minutes.

Dr. Robb made one very interesting experiment a few days ago in the interest of a large bicycle company which sent to him specimens of carbon steel and nickel steel for the purpose of having him test them with the Röntgen rays, and see if they showed any radical differences in the crystalline structure. Photographs were taken as desired, but at the time of my visit only negative results had been obtained.

Dr. Robb realizes the great desirability of finding a stronger source of Röntgen rays, and has himself begun experimenting with exhaustive bulbs made of aluminium. One of these he has already finished, and has obtained some results with it, but not such as are entirely satisfactory, owing to the great difficulty in obtaining a high vacuum without special facilities.

I also visited Professor U. I. Pupin of Columbia College, who has been making numerous experiments with the Röntgen rays, and has produced at least one very remarkable shadow picture. This is of the hand of a gentleman resident in New York, who, while on a hunting trip in England a few months ago, was so unfortunate as to discharge his gun into his right hand, no less than forty shot lodging in the palm and fingers. The hand has since healed completely; but the shot remain in it, the doctors being unable to remove them, because unable to determine their exact location. The result is that the hand is almost useless, and often painful.

Hearing of this case, Professor Pupin induced the gentleman to allow him to attempt a photograph of the hand. He used a Crookes tube. The distance from the tube to the plate was only five inches, and the hand lay between. After waiting fifty minutes the plate was examined. Not only did every bone of the hand show with beautiful distinctness, but each one of the forty shot was to be seen almost as plainly as if it lay there on the table; and, most remarkable of all, a number of shot were seen through the bones of the fingers, showing that the bones were transparent to the lead.

In making this picture, Professor Pupin excited his tube by means of a powerful Holtz machine, thus following Dr. Morton in the substitution of statical electricity for the more common induction coil.

Professor Pupin sees no reason why the whole skeleton of the human body should not be shown completely in a photograph as soon as sufficiently powerful bulbs can be obtained. He thinks that it would be possible to make Crookes tubes two feet in diameter instead of a few inches, as at present.

Thomas A. Edison has also been devoting himself, with his usual energy, to experiments with the Röntgen rays, and announces confidently that in the near future he will be able to photograph the human brain, through the heavy bones of the skull, and perhaps even to get a shadow picture showing the human skeleton through the tissues of the body.

COMMENTS ON X-RAY PSEUDOSCIENCE BY GEORGE M. STERNBERG

Published in February 1897 in the journal Science, *George M. Sternberg's article* "Science and Pseudo-Science in Medicine," *excerpted below, provides a contemporary account of dubious early medical applications of X-ray technology. Patients are described as being "under the X-ray" for periods as long as nine hours. From a modern vantage point, knowing what we do about the risks of X-ray exposure, the article shows not only how an overzealous public can be taken in by the newest medical fad but also how the full risks of new imaging technologies may not be apparent for many years after their initial application.*

"Science and Pseudo-Science in Medicine"

By George M. Sternberg

The fact that a considerable proportion of those who are sick from various acute or chronic ailments recover after a time, independently of the use of medicinal agents or methods of treatment, taken in connection with this tendency to ascribe recovery to the treatment employed, makes it an easy matter to obtain certificates of cure for any nostrum which an unprincipled money-seeker may see fit to offer to a credulous public. If ten in a thousand of those who have used the alleged remedy believe themselves to have been benefited, their certificates will answer all purposes of exploitation and the 990 will not be heard from by the general public.

As was to have been expected, the X-ray has already been made a source of revenue by more than one pseudo-scientist. The following account of the modus operandi of its supposed therapeutic action has recently been published in the newspapers:

"After the Crookes tube is excited by the coil the magnetic lines of force are projected down in the same manner as they pass off from a magnet, and traversing the intervening space, pass through the body down to the floor, and back to the coil and tube again, completing the circuit."

"The X-ray is electrostatic in character and of a very high potential. With every discharge from the Crookes tube oxygen is liberated in the body, as well as the surrounding atmosphere, which, combining with nascent oxygen, forms ozone."

"It is due to the electrolysis produced in the body that we are able to destroy the bacilli in contagious disease, ozone being the most powerful germicide known."

We remark, first, that we do not fully understand why "the magneticlines of force" are reflected back by the floor, "completing the circuit." Inasmuch as the X-rays pass through wood, this mysterious action of the floor appears to call for some further explanation. We will pass by the ingenious explanation of the formation of ozone, as a result of the action of the X-ray, to call attention to the mistaken statement that ozone is "the most powerful germicide known." Upon this point I take the liberty of quoting from the Manual of Bacteriology:

"The experiments of Frankel show that the aerobic bacteria grow abundantly in the presence of pure oxygen, and some species even more so than in ordinary air."

"*Ozone*—It was formerly supposed that ozone would prove to be a most valuable agent for disinfecting purposes, but recent experiments show that it is not so active a germicide as was anticipated, and that from a practical point of view it has comparatively little value."

"Lukaschewitsch found that one gramme in the space of a cubic metre failed to kill anthrax spores in twenty-four hours. The cholera spirillum in a moist state was killed in this time by the same amount, but fifteen hours' exposure failed to destroy it. Ozone for these experiments was developed by means of electricity."

"Wyssokowicz found that the presence of ozone in a culture medium restrained the development of the anthrax bacillus, the bacillus of typhoid fever, and others tested, but concludes that this is rather due to the oxidation of bases contained in the nutrient medium than to a direct action upon the pathogenic bacteria."

"Sonntag, in his carefully conducted experiments, in which a current of ozonized air was made to pass over silk threads to which were attached anthrax spores, had an entirely negative result. The anthrax bacillus from the spleen of a mouse, and free from spores, was then tested, also with a negative result, even after exposure to the oxonized air for twenty minutes at a time on four successive days. In another experiment several test organisms (Bacillus anthracis, Bacillus pneumoniae of Friedlander, Staphylococcus pyogenes aureus, Staphylococcus pyogenes albus, Bacillus muriseptiicus, Bacillus crassus sputigenus) were exposed on silk threads for twenty-four hours in an atmosphere containing 4.1 milligrammes of ozone to the litre of air (0.19 volumes per cent.). The result was entirely negative. When the amount was increased to 13.53 milligrammes per litre the anthrax bacillus and Staphylococcus pyogenes albus failed to grow after twenty-four hours' exposure. The conclusion reached by Nissen, from his own experiments and a careful consideration of those previously made by others, is that ozone is of no practical value as a germicide in therapeutics or disinfection."

From a practical point of view the use of the X-ray in the practice of the Chicago doctor, to whom the above quoted explanation of its therapeutic action is attributed, appears to have been quite successful. He says:

"For the last eight months I have had patients under the X-ray in my laboratory from 9 a.m. to 6 p.m., duration of treatment varying from a-half to four hours at each treatment, and not once with any bad result in any case."

Now it is evident that a physician who has patients coming to his office from 9 a.m. to 6 p.m. every day is in the enjoyment of a very handsome professional income. And if, as I imagine, many of these patients are well-dressed ladies with more leisure than judgment, they are no doubt satisfied to pay well for the opportunity of having the latest scientific treatment applied to their cases and to await their turn in the anteroom of this distinguished "professor of electro-therapeutics." The article from which we have quoted, and which appears to answer all the purposes of a free advertisement, concludes as follows:

"It must not be forgotten that electric phenomena are very powerful, and not every man who can buy a machine is capable of applying it. The electric machine must be as skillfully adjusted to each individual as the microscope to a specimen submitted to it. It is a treatment full of danger if ignorantly or rashly handled, but beyond price in value to the skilled and careful electro-therapeutist."

We do not propose to prejudge the question of the possible therapeutic value of the X-ray, but we think it safe to predict that it will not be found of any value for the destruction of pathogenic bacteria in the tissues, inasmuch as it has been shown by several competent observers to have very little, if any, germicidal action; and because there is no experimental evidence which justifies the belief that these low vegetable organisms can be destroyed by any physical or chemical agents which would not at the same time destroy the vitality of the less resistant cellular elements of the tissues. If time permitted I might further illustrate the temporary successes of recent pseudo-scientific discoveries by referring to the "cryptococous xanthogenicus" of Domingos Freire, of Brazil, the Bacillus malarise of Klebs and Tomasi Crudelli, etc., etc. The spectacle of a learned clergyman, supplied by nature with a brain and a pair of lungs, sitting day after day with an "electropoise" attached to his leg for the purpose of "taking on oxygen freely from the atmosphere" recalls the "blue grass craze" of twenty-five years ago.

PEOPLE V. YUM

The following excerpt is taken from a court opinion ordered by the Court of Appeal of the State of California, Fourth Appellate District, Division Two, in the case of

People v. Yum *(2003). The defendant and appellant, Paul Seong Chul Yum, had been convicted of two counts of second-degree murder, but his case was appealed, in part on the grounds that the court "erred by not permitting evidence of the defendant's SPECT [Single Photon Computed Tomography] brain scan" as evidence for a mental disorder, post-traumatic stress disorder (PTSD). The opinion of the Court of Appeal represents an early and interesting ruling on the admissibility of functional imaging of the brain as evidence. Footnotes have been omitted.*

Dr. Daniel G. Amen, of the Amen Clinic for Behavioral Medicine, performed a SPECT brain scan on defendant. "Brain SPECT imaging" is described on Dr. Amen's website as "a nuclear medicine study that uses very small doses of radioisotopes to evaluate brain blood flow and activity patterns. SPECT is widely recognized as an effective tool for evaluating brain function in strokes, seizures, dementia and head trauma. . . . During the past 11 years our clinics have developed this technology further to evaluate and subtype ADD, anxiety and depression, aggression, the effects of substance abuse, and non-responsive neuropsychiatric conditions."

At the Evidence Code section 402 hearing on the prosecution's motion to exclude the brain scan and Dr. Amen's testimony, Dr. Amen testified that defendant's brain scan showed results associated with trauma and consistent with the SPECT pattern found in other PTSD sufferers. He also testified that SPECT is typically used to diagnose brain trauma, strokes, seizures, and dementia but not psychiatric disorders.

In support of its motion, the prosecution presented articles from medical journals indicating brain imaging has been deemed scientifically acceptable to diagnose stroke, epilepsy, brain tumors, dementia, and Alzheimer's disease, and movement disorders, like Parkinson's disease. The same articles also question the use of SPECT to diagnose psychiatric disorders. The prosecution's expert witness, Dr. Peter Conti, testified there are three approved clinical uses for SPECT: the diagnosis of stroke, epilepsy or seizure, and dementia. Other applications are experimental and the use of SPECT to diagnose brain trauma and PTSD is controversial. In this particular case, Dr. Conti disagreed that defendant's SPECT scans showed abnormalities.

The court ruled the defense had not shown SPECT has achieved general scientific acceptance and therefore the SPECT evidence was not admissible.

Where expert testimony is based on the application of a new scientific technique, its proponent must demonstrate that the method employed is reliable—that is, the particular technique or test must have gained general acceptance in the field to which it belongs. The trial court's ruling on this issue is subject to independent review by the appellate court.

Defendant contends that the proffered testimony of Dr. Amen was not subject at all to Kelly [a previous California Supreme Court ruling that evidence based on a new scientific technique is only admissible on showing general acceptance of the technique in the scientific community] because it was expert medical opinion and thus fell outside the realm of evidence considered a "new scientific technique." This contention is belied by the record.

As demonstrated in the evidentiary hearing, the proffered evidence was that of Dr. Amen describing brain SPECT imaging and his methods pertaining thereto, and opining that the scan revealed diminished activity in defendant's left temporal lobe, and hyperactivity elsewhere, findings consistent with brain trauma and correlated with violence, anger, and aggression. Clearly, the purpose of Dr. Amen's testimony was to put forth evidence of defendant's SPECT scan in an attempt to show he had temporal lobe damage caused by brain trauma, which in turn caused him to kill his mother and sister. Accordingly, in order for Dr. Amen's testimony to be admissible, defendant had to demonstrate that the use of SPECT scan imaging to diagnose brain trauma and PTSD was generally accepted in the field of brain imaging and neurology. Defendant failed to make this showing.

In order to establish general acceptance of the use of SPECT scans to diagnose brain trauma and PTSD, defendant had to show substantial agreement among a cross-section of the relevant scientific community. Defendant had to demonstrate a consensus in the field, which Dr. Amen's testimony did not. Our review of the testimony of Doctors Amen and Conti and the pertinent medical literature reveals that the majority of qualified members in the neurology and brain imaging community does not support the use of SPECT scans to diagnose prior head trauma and mental disorders like PTSD and considers the technique generally unreliable for this purpose. Accordingly, we hold the trial court properly excluded Dr. Amen's testimony.

PAUL C. LAUTERBUR'S NOBEL PRIZE LECTURE

The following is the lecture delivered by Dr. Paul C. Lauterbur upon being awarded the 2003 Nobel Prize for Medicine and Physiology in recognition of his groundbreaking discovery, magnetic resonance imaging. The lecture recounts his somewhat unlikely path toward the discovery, of which he exclaims "All detours should be so productive!"

"All Science Is Interdisciplinary—From Magnetic Moments to Molecules to Men"

Nobel Lecture, December 8, 2003
By Paul C. Lauterbur

Biomedical Magnetic Resonance Laboratory, University of Illinois, Urbana, IL 61801, USA.

The title is not a tribute to some trendy hybrid field, but an introduction to a lecture on a Nobel Prize for Physiology or Medicine that is shared by a chemist and a physicist.

Few events could illustrate more clearly the blending both at the boundaries, and sometimes through the bodies, of our disciplines. For that is what they are, disciplines, not natural categories with rigid boundaries to be defended against intrusions, but guides to instruction and efficient administration.

Historically, the record is clear. Chemistry, for example, was cobbled together from mystical alchemy, metallurgy, physics, mineralogy, medicine, and cookery, eliminating incompatibilities as it evolved and consolidated into a more-or-less unified discipline. Physics has been formed, and enriched, by contributions from astronomy, mechanics, mathematics, chemistry, and other sciences. We have recently observed the rationalization of much of biology by chemistry, with the help of physics.

Nuclear magnetic resonance began within physics, at a confluence among particle physics, condensed matter physics, spectroscopy, and electromagnetics. Discovery of ways to observe the subtle properties of atomic nuclei in solids, liquids, and eventually gases, earned Felix Bloch and Edward Purcell a Nobel Prize in Physics in 1952. Applications to studies of molecular motions and structures began almost immediately. The discoverers themselves, it is told, even used their own bodies as samples. In an early predecessor to MRI, Jay Singer measured blood flow in a human arm, and actual medical measurements were started when Erich Odeblad, a Swedish M.D., constructed apparatus and devised methods to study very small quantities of human secretions for medical purposes. Other biological studies followed, in other labs, using animal tissues, including hearts, and entire small animals.

In 1971, Raymond Damadian observed that some malignant tissue, obtained from implanted tumors removed from rats, had longer NMR [nuclear magnetic resonance] relaxation times than many normal tissues. This observation caught the attention of several people, and Hollis decided to attempt to confirm and extend it by a study of a related system, Morris hepatomas in rats, readily available to him at Johns Hopkins University. At one point, a post-doctoral fellow in his laboratory, Leon Saryan, brought some of the animals to the small company in western Pennsylvania which had actually carried out the earlier Damadian work. There, the rats were sacrificed and dissected and the tissue sample studied by NMR. I happened to be present to observe the entire process, for reasons described elsewhere, and, as a chemist not ordinarily involved with animal experiments, found them rather distasteful. All such NMR experiments were subject to error from non-uniformities in sample composition, the static magnetic field, and the radiofrequency magnetic field. However, the differences in the NMR signals from one tissue to another, normal as well as diseased, seemed robust in the experiments I observed. I thought they might actually be reproducible and useful, especially if the signal intensities, relaxation times, etc., could be measured from outside the living body with sufficient spatial resolution.

That evening, over dinner, it occurred to me that, as the frequencies of NMR signals depended on the local magnetic field, there might be a general way to locate them in a non-uniform magnetic field. I knew, however, that a static field could not have a unique value in each location in three dimensions, but that a complex shape could be represented by an expansion in a set of functions such as those provided by the correction, or "shim" fields, available on NMR machines to cancel unwanted magnetic field non-uniformities, term by term, with linear gradients, quadratic ones, etc. Could this be the answer? A little reflection made me doubt it. I recalled that single-center expansions of molecular wave-functions had been tried in quantum chemistry, but converged on useful solutions slowly and poorly. An alternative occurred to me. What if one used a large set of simple linear gradients, oriented in many directions in turn in three dimensions? I knew of no examples in any field. This was early September 1971, and X-ray CT [computed tomography] was not yet widely known, and neither had I encountered the similar ideas that were being tested in radioastronomy by Bracewell and in electron microscopy by Herman and Gordon, and by others in different fields. Nor did I know of any mathematics to solve such problems, but I recalled another idea from quantum chemistry, that when equations were not solvable in analytic form, an iterative method, in which approximate solutions were compared to known properties and systematically adjusted to a closer and closer fit, could be used.

To test this idea, I wrote down small arrays of numbers such as 1s and 0s, in small arrays 4×4 or even 8×8 square, and added them along the vertical and horizontal directions, representing the 1-dimensional data that would be generated by linear magnetic field gradients perpendicular to those directions, as well as data, at 45° and 135°, that could be generated similarly. The "data" could then be "back-projected" across the image space as a series of bands and summed where they crossed, from which the trial image of summed intensities could be projected in each of the original directions for comparison with the actual "data," and modified by added or multiplicative terms to agree with it. The procedure might then be repeated, in hopes that the next computed trial image would be a closer approximation on each cycle to the synthetic original one. I asked local mathematicians whether such a procedure was known and would work. All said they knew of no examples, and some said it was obviously valid, while others said it was clear that it would not converge, so I just tried it myself, with pencil and paper calculations. The result, with such simple mathematical "phantoms" (test objects) at least, was that the calculations converged very rapidly indeed. Later, a computer scientist with whom I had consulted came across a paper in a subsequent issue of a journal that used exactly my algorithm. This simultaneously validated the method and eliminated my claims to priority. I later learned that much work on the so-called "reconstruction from projections" problem had been published, by many people in many contexts, in recent years, almost all developed independently in different fields. My real interest, however, was in the magnetic resonance imaging problem, and that remained unique.

I then turned my attention to the question of whether there would be enough NMR signal-to-noise ratio with large enough radiofrequency coils to surround a human body and the low magnetic fields I thought might be practical in resistive magnets over such large volumes. The standard reference, "Nuclear Magnetism," by Abragam provided equations that suggested that the answer was favorable. At about the same time, my review of the magnet literature revealed that resistive magnets with fields of the order of 1000 gauss (0.1 tesla) and diameters of about 1 meter could be constructed and operated economically with enough field uniformity to support the NMR experiments I had in mind.

It then appeared that all the requirements could be met if the right research and development could be done, so that a new and useful medical diagnostic tool would be available. But first, there was another matter to resolve. A patent attorney at the company had advised me to do no experiments at my university, as they would compromise my patent position. He and I had been actively working on preparing patent application documents, in exchange for his fee of a percentage of any financial returns that might result. Unfortunately, a business dispute developed between us in connection with the company, and he declined to continue with our agreement. When that happened, I made a patent disclosure to my university, which in turn sent it to the organization they used to evaluate such documents and prepare patent applications.

In the meantime, I began experiments, preparing test objects by attaching 1 mm diameter glass melting point capillaries to the inside of 5 mm glass NMR sample tubes, the capillaries filled with ordinary water (H_2O) and the outer tubes with heavy water (D_2O). The reason for the D_2O was to roughly match the magnetic susceptibility across the sample so that the capillary signals would be less distorted than they would have been with air in that space. I first tried three capillaries, but the signals were too complex for easy interpretation, so I tried just two. I also tried using the linear gradients in the magnetic field supplied by the appropriate "shim" controls on a small analytical NMR spectrometer in the Chemistry Department, with 5 mm sample tubes filled with ordinary water. As expected, their projections were half-ellipses, or semi-circles for the proper adjustment of the strength of the gradient. For an actual test of the image mathematics on real data, I attached a paper disc, marked at intervals of 45°, to the outer tube containing two capillaries and rotated it to orientations of 0°, 45°, 90° and 135° relative to the gradient direction while recording the NMR signal on a pen and ink recorder. I then digitized the recordings by measuring the height of the curves at intervals with a ruler and recording the numbers on a piece of paper, with the intervals corresponding to the projections of a square grid at each angle. The numbers were then transferred manually to punch cards that could be fed to a reader attached to the departmental instrument control computer, originally intended only to operate an X-ray diffractometer for single crystal structure determinations. Its memory (ferrite cores) was so limited that all calculations had to be made in integer ("fixed point") mode, and intermediate results had to be punched out on a deck of cards to be reentered later for the next step, and each subprogram had to be kept on a separate deck of punched cards. The final result was then printed by a typewriter as a

20 × 20 array of numbers, and the "image" produced by hand-drawn contours on that array. This seems tedious on later description but was exciting then because the whole process and its results were being encountered for the first time, especially as I recognized that the "pictures" were a new kind of image, based on principles completely different from those behind other imaging methods. To emphasize this point, I coined the new word "zeugmatography" as a description, checking with a classical scholar for its fidelity to ancient roots and with a speaker of contemporary Greek to ensure that the meaning of "zeugma" had not shifted during later centuries.

Reassured, I used it in a manuscript I wrote for the journal *Nature*, which was summarily rejected. I felt this was a mistake, not because I foresaw all of the medical applications that would follow, but because of the physical uniqueness of the concept. I was also trying to think of another example that would work in practice, but it was to be over a quarter of a century later that an example, involving the differential shift of the spectra of two closely spaced atoms by an inhommogeous electric field, was published, but the authors did not notice the similarities. My appeal to *Nature* was followed by submission of a revised version of my manuscript containing references to cancer and other more obviously relevant topics, and this time it was accepted. Almost thirty years later, *Nature* publicly celebrated its appearance there. Slightly earlier, I had presented my results in a short contributed paper at an American Physical Society meeting, which then had a policy of accepting any meeting talk by a member, but it was attended by only a handful of listeners, one of whom was a graduate student who told me that his professor had done the same thing, but I never found any evidence that he had. A similar pattern repeated itself several times in later years, with people telling me that they had the same ideas but had not followed them up with experiments and publication.

This work, and its subsequent elaborations, became the subject of my lectures afterward at most meetings I attended, including seminars. Before I began describing it in detail everywhere, however, the University's agent rejected the patent application because they felt that it could not generate enough funds to pay for the application process. I then asked my university for permission to pursue the application independently but never received a reply. I was not in a financial position to quit my job and defy the university, and the grace period for applying for a U.S. patent after publication had nearly expired, so I abandoned that idea and decided instead to encourage others to pursue this new technology, inviting everyone interested to visit my laboratory to observe our efforts and learn from us. People did come, from industry, academia, and government laboratories, foreign and domestic, and I began supplying a bibliography of such work to all and helping to organize meetings on the subject to compare our methods and results. Among these were Professor Raymond Andrew and members of his group at Nottingham University, and Drs. Mansfield, Moore, and others there, as well as representatives of medical instrument companies and medical doctors and medical physicists themselves. As I hoped, interest began building as many other groups were involved.

We continued our work, which shortly involved graduate students and postdoctoral fellows as well as undergraduate research students, and, as I had hoped, more contributions were published by other laboratories, with some remarkable early images from Waldo Hinshaw in Andrew's group at Nottingham. As the depth and breadth of application grew, both large and small companies began to see opportunities, and within less than ten years commercial instruments began to come to market, large enough to hold a human being and to support true clinical research. Competitive pressures among physicians, industrial interest, and multiplying applications and techniques began to generate the explosive growth that was to characterize the past twenty years, leading, among other things, to the recognition of this phenomenon by the Royal Swedish Academy of Sciences. I and my group continued to make contributions through this period as well, some of them significant, but the most gratifying experiences emotionally were those when a stranger would volunteer "you saved my daughter's life," or "your machine saved me from an unnecessary operation." By the end of the millennium, despite the continuing excitement of the field, almost thirty years of a detour from chemistry to medical imaging began to pall, and I changed my focus to a field of chemical research, just in time for my past to catch up with me in the form of a Nobel Prize. All detours should be so productive!

Source: ©The Nobel Foundation 2003.

Electromagnetic Radiation and the Atom

A summary of the characteristics of the imaging technologies currently in use are presented in Table B.1. The physical principles by which the different modalities interact with matter are discussed in the following section.

ELECTROMAGNETIC RADIATION AND THE ATOM

The purpose of this section is to briefly explain at an intuitive level the interactions of atoms with the forms of electromagnetic energy used for medical imaging. The discovery and application of the imaging technologies thus can be developed with a minimum of the physics included here.

All forms of imaging use some kind of radiated energy to produce a picture that can be interpreted by physicians. This energy can be projected from either the outside (X-rays, ultrasound, magnetic resonance imaging [MRI]) or emitted from inside during radioisotope imaging (positron emission tomography [PET], single photon computed tomography [SPECT]). To understand how the different modalities of medical imaging produce an image, it is important to know what energy is and how it can be harnessed and released. Learning about the structure of the atom and how it interacts with radiation helps us understand how medical imaging works, as well as some of its limitations and potential dangers if misused. The pioneers of X-rays were hampered by not understanding how the mysterious "light" was produced and how it interacted with matter. Had more been appreciated about how X-rays interacted with matter, far fewer unknowing researchers would have become martyrs to harmful overexposure to the miraculous rays.

A RADIATION PRIMER

All of the imaging modalities, except for ultrasound, employ one form or another of electromagnetic radiation. The specific type of radiation involved

Table B.1 Summary of Imaging Modalities

Imaging modality	Transmission X-ray	Fluoroscopic X-ray	Computed tomography	Nuclear imaging (SPECT/PET)	Ultrasound	MRI
Radiation	X-ray	X-ray	X-ray	Gamma Ray	Ultrasound	Radio frequency
Soft tissue contrast	Weak	Weak	High	Moderate/high	Moderate	High
Detector	Film	Image intensifier	Solid state	Scintillation camera	Piezo crystal	Coil antenna
Resolution	High	Moderate	High	Low	Low	High
Anatomy (A) Physiology (P)	A	A	A	P	A and P	A and P
Cost	Lowest	Low	High	Moderate	Low	Highest

determines what will show up in an image. That means that the same field of view may look different depending on the kind of electromagnetic radiation used. For example, X-ray images will show up bone clearly, while muscle and fat will be more noticeable than bone in a magnetic resonance image. Physicians choose the imaging method to highlight the physiological or anatomical system they suspect to be malfunctioning.

Images are formed from the interaction of radiation with an object. A simple image is a shadow on which an object blocks the passage of the radiation by reflection or absorption. The word "radiation" is used here in its most general sense. Radiation is energy that travels through space or matter. This includes X-rays, radio waves, sound, heat, and visible light. Two types of radiation commonly employed in medicine are electromagnetic radiation and particle radiation. Particle radiation, such as streams of protons, electrons, or neutrons, is not used for medical imaging and we will only touch on it here. Because the particles interact strongly with matter, they do not travel far in tissues before being absorbed. Depending on their energy, the particles can damage cellular structure and this is put to use in therapy to kill tumor cells. The highest energy electromagnetic radiation can be used in a similar therapeutic fashion. The imaging modalities we will consider (again excepting ultrasound) use either low-energy (nonionizing) radiation or carefully metered high-energy ionizing radiation to reduce tissue damage. Radiation dosage is carefully monitored to minimize risk to both the patient and health care personnel.

Ultrasound imaging utilizes a nonelectromagnetic radiation form of energy to reveal inner structures. Sound waves are transmitted only in a matter medium—solid, liquid, or gas. By contrast, radiative energy (electromagnetic radiation) can travel through the vacuum of space. The Sun's radiative heat, light, and cosmic rays travel through a vacuum in space to reach the Earth. In the absence of a material medium, such as air, sound waves do not exist. Two galaxies colliding in space produce no sound.

We experience interaction with electromagnetic radiation every day and everywhere we go. Many kinds of electromagnetic radiation are familiar, even though we may not recognize them as deriving from the same source, the movement of electric charge, and the associated magnetic fields. Heat (long wavelength infrared radiation) from a fire warms us, and shorter wavelength infrared light guards homes or changes the television channel. Radio and television provide entertainment, cell phones and wireless Internet routers connect people, RADAR warns against aircraft collisions and enforces the speed limit on highways, microwave ovens cook food, and visible light aids in reading these words. Ultraviolet rays (UVB, UVC) can provide a suntan, although they can also cause skin cancer. Other forms of electromagnetic radiation are less familiar but also are part of our lives. Moderate energy X-rays reveal the inside of the body as ghostly shadows on photographic film and fluoroscopes or as a three-dimensional tomographic image CT scan. High energy X-rays and gamma rays are used to selectively kill fast-growing cancer cells, although high doses damage healthy cells.

Although many people do not make the connection from low to high energy, all these forms of electromagnetic radiation are related to one another (see Figure B.1). Scientists often think of all of these forms of electromagnetic energy as waves traveling through the vacuum of space at the same speed, the speed of light (186,000 miles/second or 300,000 kilometers/second). The amount of energy carried by each kind of electromagnetic wave is related to its frequency and the number of wave crests per second (see Figure B.2). A drummer tapping slowly (low frequency) on a drumhead expends less energy than when she is beating a fast (high frequency) drum roll. According to Albert Einstein's theory of relativity, energy and matter (particle mass) are freely interconvertible when that mass is traveling near the speed of light. So, under some circumstances, the radiation acts like it is a wave, and other times like it is a particle called a photon. A photon travels at the speed of light and does not have any mass, because it has been transformed into pure energy.

It is easiest to visualize photons as the way electromagnetic radiation interacts with matter. Sunlight interacting with an object and reflecting back to our eyes can be as direct as a red apple absorbing the photons with the energy of green light, or as complex as the wave-like interference patterns that produce the false colors of a peacock tail feather. As you may have noticed among the types of electromagnetic radiation, ultraviolet light, X-ray, and gamma-ray photons are energetic enough to cause damage to tissues (see the bar in Figure B.1). Because photons with these energies are so powerful, they can disrupt the bonds holding atoms together in the molecules that allow the body to function. What do these photons interact with? To answer that, a brief discussion about the anatomy of an atom is needed.

ATOMIC STRUCTURE 101

An atom is the smallest piece of an element that reacts chemically like that element. Elements have different properties, ranging from hydrogen (a gas) to iron (a metal), which join in different proportions with each other to produce molecules that further combine to substances and objects that we recognize. Atoms are tiny, nearly ten thousand times smaller than the wavelength of visible light. In turn, the atom is made up of still smaller parts (see Figure B.3). At its core is an extremely dense positively charged nucleus containing protons (heavy positively charged particles) and neutrons (heavy uncharged particles) surrounded by a cloud of light (1/1,837th the mass of a proton) negatively charged electrons. The number of protons, neutrons, and electrons in an atom is determined by the identity of the element. An atom is almost entirely empty space. The nucleus occupies only one-millionth of a millionth of the volume of the atom. Many of the interactions of electromagnetic radiation occur with the atom's electrons. Because the electron orbits extend out

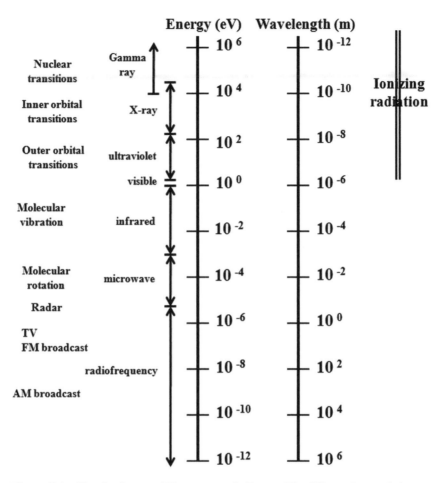

Figure B.1 The Continuum of Electromagnetic Energy. The different forms of electro-magnetic energy arranged according to their increasing energy. The energy level at which damage to tissue occurs is indicated by the double line. Since all electromagnetic radiation travels at the speed of light (186,000 miles/second or 300,000 kilometers/second), the amount of energy a photon carries depends on the frequency (wave cycles per second).

far beyond the nucleus, it is the electrons that contact the world and determine how atoms interact with each other (chemistry) to form chemical compounds that assemble to form rocks, hot dogs, and people.

Besides interacting with energy from the outside, certain forms of elements are unstable and break down to produce atomic fragments or release electromagnetic energy. The number of protons in the nucleus of an atom defines the element while the number of neutrons plus the number of protons in the nucleus defines an isotope. Isotopes of an element act chemically identical to

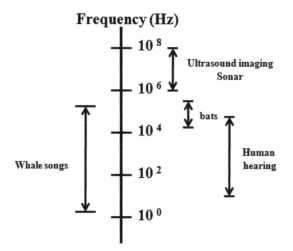

Figure B.2   Wavelength and frequency of sound spectrum.

one another, although the nuclei are different, because the atoms have the same number and arrangement of electrons. Multiple isotopes can have the same element depending on how many neutrons are present in each. The nucleus has a complex internal structure of its own, which reflects the relative numbers of neutrons and protons and determines its relative stability. Out of the 2,500 or so isotopes of the elements, only 270 are stable, and the nuclei do not change over time. The rest of the isotopic nuclei are unstable to various degrees and break down, producing photons of different types. They produce these photons at characteristic rates by a process termed "radioactive decay," which is important in providing "light from the inside" for SPECT and PET imaging. The nuclear structure of isotopes plays a role in the magnetic properties of atomic nuclei, which is important for MRI.

So, how do electromagnetic radiation and the components of the atom interact? The following section will outline the processes that are the basis for medical imaging.

INTERACTION OF RADIATION WITH ATOMS

The positively charged nucleus of an atom holds on tightly to the electrons surrounding it. In 1913, the Danish physicist Niels Bohr proposed a structure for the atom that placed the electrons in orbits or levels around the nucleus, much like a miniature solar system. Although this is not an exact picture of an atom, and more precise quantum mechanical descriptions are available, it is a simple heuristic device to explain many things about how atoms interact with electromagnetic and particle radiation and with each other.

In Bohr's model (see Figure B.3), the electron orbits are arranged in concentric layers outward from the nucleus, with each level or orbital further

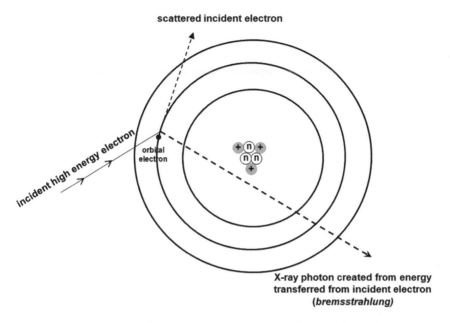

Figure B.3 Bohr Model of the Atom. In this model, the light negatively charged electrons orbit a heavy positively charged nucleus. An analogous model for the nucleus defines energy levels within the nucleus. These models are sufficient to describe the interaction of radiation with the atom but neither is an accurate physical description because at the dimensions and energies of the atom the classical physics of everyday objects must be replaced by quantum mechanical descriptions to accurately portray the system.

away from the nucleus of higher energy. Quantum theory states that electrons can only move between levels if (1) there is a vacancy, and (2) they absorb or give up exactly enough energy to match the difference between the two levels. X-rays used for medical imaging are generated when an electron freed from another atom and traveling at a high enough speed (remember a high speed particle is one form of energy) passes very close to or collides with an orbital electron. Since both the orbital and colliding electron are negatively charged, they repel one another. Most interactions result in the colliding electron being deflected from the orbital cloud of electrons, transferring a portion of the energy from its high speed (kinetic energy) to the orbital electron, which then releases a photon corresponding to the amount of kinetic energy absorbed, a process called **bremsstrahlung**. If the energy of the impinging electron is sufficiently high, the emitted photon's energy is in the X-ray range. Much less frequently, because the atom is mostly empty space, the inbound electron hits the bull's-eye, knocking the bound orbital electron free from the atom. There is now a vacancy in that electron shell. Like a boulder rolling down hill, an electron from an orbital shell further from the nucleus drops down to the lower energy orbital, giving up the energy difference between the starting and final levels as a photon. An electron orbital closer to the positively charged nucleus is higher energy, thus the released photon's energy can be captured in the X-ray range if an inner orbital is involved.

THE PRODUCTION OF MEDICAL X-RAYS

The larger the number of positively charged protons in the nucleus, the tighter the negatively charged electrons are held in their orbitals, and the more energy is released by an impinging high-speed electron. X-rays are defined as having energies greater than 100 electron volts (eV) (1 eV = the energy imparted to an electron traveling through an electrical potential of 1 volt). In a modern X-ray tube generator, electrons are released from metal atoms in a metal wire filament (negatively charged cathode) by heating in a chamber from which air and other gasses are pumped, producing a vacuum. The vacuum is necessary to prevent the free electrons from reacting with those molecules. The free electrons are concentrated and accelerated to high speed in an electrical field on the order of 50,000–120,000 volts (50–120 kilovolts [kV]) and allowed to crash into a positively charged target (anode) that is made of, or coated with, an element chosen to produce X-rays of the desired energy, which depends on the application. This process is triggered for only a brief fraction of a second while the exposure is being made and then the current is shut down; otherwise, the tube components would be damaged from the extreme heat. The elements most often used to generate X-rays for medical imaging are the metals molybdenum (17,500 eV [or 17.5 keV, where 1 keV = 1,000 eV]), rhodium (20.2 keV), and tungsten (59.3 keV). The nucleus of each of these metals contains many protons (42, 45, and 74, respectively), holding the electrons tightly to the atom. Taking X-ray images of steel boilers to spot welding flaws requires higher X-ray energies than biological tissue, although the principles remain the same.

X-rays are absorbed or scattered most efficiently by elements with many protons and neutrons in their nuclei. The body is made mostly of elements with small numbers of protons in their nuclei, including hydrogen (1), carbon (6), nitrogen (7), oxygen (8), phosphorus (15), and sulfur (16). Moderately high-energy X-rays, termed "diagnostic X-rays," such as those produced from molybdenum, rhodium, and tungsten are absorbed only slightly or scattered in many parts of the body, producing a faint haze on radiographic film. Different tissues absorb diagnostic X-rays generally related to their water (hydrogen) content. Calcium, with 20 protons in its nucleus and 20 electrons in its orbitals, is an exception. It binds its electrons tightly enough to scatter significant amounts of X-rays, so bones, which are largely composed of calcium, show up clearly in an X-ray photograph. So do many foreign metal objects such as surgical screws, safety pins, bullets, and other items. Muscle, fat, cartilage, and connective tissue absorb intermediate amounts of X-rays, producing images that, although largely unintelligible to the average viewer, can be interpreted by skilled radiologists.

GAMMA-RAY IMAGING

Another form of electromagnetic radiation, gamma rays, is very much like X-rays, except that these rays have even higher energy and they are produced by a different process. Gamma rays for medical imaging come from spontaneous changes in the internal structure of an unstable atomic nucleus, giving rise to photon emission. Atomic nuclei have energy levels analogous to electronic energy levels of the whole atom that produce X-rays upon high-energy electron bombardment. Natural radioisotopes of lead, bismuth, thallium, radium, thorium, and actinium exist, some of which were used for biological studies to "trace" the uptake and movement in biological systems started in 1911 by George Hevesy. Irène and Frédéric Joliot-Curie were awarded a Nobel Prize in 1934 for creating radioactivity by bombarding nonradioactive elements with high-energy α-particles. Some of these "artificial radioisotopes," iodine, phosphorus, and sodium, were elements more congenial to use in biological systems than the "natural" radioisotopes. They were considered "artificial" isotopes because they do not exist (other than perhaps fleetingly in the interior of stars) in nature. Ernest Lawrence's invention of the cyclotron provided another pathway. He accelerated neutrons to crash into nonradioactive elements and produced eighteen biologically useful isotopes. The cleavage (fission) of uranium nuclei when bombarded by neutrons described by Otto Hahn and Lise Meitner in 1939 would be harnessed first to produce an atomic bomb and later to produce nuclear energy in atomic reactors.

Analysis of these experiments provided the foundation for the concept of nuclear stability and the process of radioactive decay of a nucleus. During radioactive decay, a higher energy unstable nucleus is converted to a lower energy and more stable state, thus releasing photons of different types. Gamma-ray photons arise from transitions between energy states of the nucleus rather than interactions with the electron cloud outside of the nucleus used most often to produce X-rays. The energy difference is given off in part as photons of an energy characteristic of the element and isotope. X-rays can be produced by certain nuclear transitions, depending on the element and isotope, but these isotopes usually are avoided in nuclear imaging because their decay pathway is complex and gives rise to unwanted forms of radiation that are not useful for imaging.

Instead of shining gamma rays onto the subject and recording those that pass through the subject to create an X-ray image, a small amount of molecules containing a radioactive source of gamma rays are introduced into the subject. The emitted gamma photons are then collected in a detector. Because high-energy gamma rays hardly interact with body constituents, the relatively unperturbed photons travel out of the body in straight lines, which allows their point of origin in the body such as the liver or brain to be calculated. Thus, gamma-ray imaging is fundamentally different from X-ray imaging in that no anatomical structure, only the position of the emitted photon, is determined. A selection of carrier molecules to which the radioactive isotopes can be attached governs where in the body the isotope is retained. This provides specificity and flexibility as well as the ability to monitor specific functional processes. The isotopes used for gamma-ray imaging are chosen for the energy of gamma-photon emission, half-life, and lack of emissions of additional ionizing short-range radiation (alpha, beta) during their decay, which would expose the subject to tissue damage near the source of the radiation.

Currently, two versions of gamma-ray medical imaging are used, known by their acronyms, SPECT and PET. They differ by the decay mode of the particular radioisotope used. Both technologies utilize special cameras instead of film and apply image reconstruction techniques to provide three-dimensional localization of the source of the radiation. SPECT employs a camera containing single-crystal elements of sodium iodide (NaI) that emit a tiny flash of light when struck by a gamma ray. Modern gamma cameras can localize where on the crystal each of the thousands of light flashes per second occurs, and a computer calculates where in the subject the gamma ray must have originated to create an image. Because of their high energy, gamma rays, like X-rays, are difficult to focus, so multiple lead collimator tubes are used to absorb stray off-axis gamma rays so that only gamma-ray photons directly beneath the camera hit the NaI crystal. This results in low sensitivity (often greater than 99.95 percent loss) and some error in localizing the source of the gamma rays producing relatively fuzzy images. Seventy percent of all radionuclide imaging studies are carried out with the metastable isotope technetium-99m (^{99m}Tc).

An improvement in resolution is provided by PET, which takes advantage of a peculiar decay mode of a number of nuclear isotopes. The unstable configurations of radioactive nuclei decay to more stable configurations by several different processes depending on the element and isotope. Certain radioisotopes, which include carbon-11, nitrogen-13, oxygen-15, fluorine-18, and rubidium-82, are present in or compatible with biological materials. These isotopes decay by the emission of a positron rather than a gamma ray. More than 80 percent of clinical PET studies are with fluorine-18, usually incorporated into fluorodeoxyglucose (FDG) for metabolism studies.

A positron ($\beta+$) is the antiparticle of the electron ($\beta-$). Matter and antimatter cannot coexist, so after traveling a fraction of a millimeter, the emitted positron encounters an electron and the two particles annihilate each other producing two very high-energy gamma-ray photons (each of energy 511 keV) traveling in exactly opposite directions (180 degrees) from each other. These photons strike NaI crystal detectors that operate on the same basic principle as those used for SPECT. New highly efficient bismuth-germanate

(BGO) crystal scintillators produce 2,500 photons of light for every 511 keV photon. Some loss of resolution results from uncertainty over where the gamma ray strikes the crystal, because at these energies, they travel some 7.5 mm within the crystal before they interact to produce light. In PET, the detectors are placed on opposite sides of the subject, and the electronics are designed to register only those photons that arrive at the same time. Coincidence detection of the two photons 180 degrees apart eliminates the need for clunky collimators with their associated loss of photons because any noncoincident signals will have originated in different decay events and are rejected by the electronics. By drawing a mathematical line between the two detectors, recording coincident events, and registering those events from multiple angles, under the best of circumstances, the source of the decay can be localized to within 0.5 cm in three dimensions in the subject. In reality, particularly for SPECT, the resolution (smallest feature that can be detected) is frequently >0.8 cm. This is due to compromises required to reduce variation across the image caused by limitations on the amount of isotope that can be safely used in patients, scan time, the number of counts accumulated per scan, and the maximum count rate for the detector.

An advantage of using PET isotopes is that they have short half-lives, meaning that they will rapidly decay and no longer be a source of radiation, thus reducing patient and personnel exposure. The four major PET isotopes for clinical imaging are oxygen-18 ($t_{1/2}$ = 2.03 minutes), carbon-11 ($t_{1/2}$ = 20.4 minutes), fluorine-18 ($t_{1/2}$ = 110 minutes), and nitrogen-13 ($t_{1/2}$ = 10 minutes). Their rapid decay, however, also means that the isotopes have to be generated close to their point of use, which requires an instrument called a cyclotron. This limits PET use mainly to major hospitals or urban centers that can support an on-site cyclotron.

MAGNETIC RESONANCE

Within an atom, both electrons and the nucleus have electrical properties that determine their interaction with each other and other atoms in their neighborhood through their electrical and magnetic fields. Wherever there is moving charge there are associated electrical and magnetic fields. This is the principle that powers an electromagnet and allows an electric motor to operate. The reverse, moving a conductor such as a wire in a magnetic field, generates an electrical current (electricity), which is the principle behind electricity generation on a wind farm, or at a hydroelectric, coal-, oil-, or gas-fired power station. In biological tissue, which is mostly water, the magnetic fields generated by each atom are difficult to observe directly, so indirect methods are necessary.

An atom's magnetic field is generated primarily by an electrical property called spin by physicists. Like an iron bar magnet, the magnetism has a direction (arbitrarily named ''North'' and South'' poles pointed in a particular direction) and thus is called a magnetic dipole. The electrons of an atom normally are paired such that their spins cancel out. Unpaired electrons do have a net magnetic dipole, and atoms or molecules harboring an unpaired electron (radicals) can be observed by electron paramagnetic resonance (EPR). They are generally highly chemically reactive, rushing to pair up their electrons by combining with a nearby atom. EPR is not widely used in medical imaging.

The protons and neutrons together in an atom's nucleus create a magnetic dipole, also called a magnetic moment because it has both a magnitude and a direction. The proton and the neutron have their own magnetic moments caused by their individual spin properties. Even though the neutron is an electrically neutral particle, the subnuclear scale internal structure of the neutron causes it to have a magnetic moment, which is opposite in direction and nearly the same magnitude to that of the proton. This gives rise to the pairing phenomenon: if (# proton + # neutrons) = even, then that nucleus has essentially no net magnetic moment. The most abundant molecule in the body is water with two hydrogens and a single oxygen atom. Fortunately for nuclear MRI, the most abundant isotope of hydrogen is ^{1}H (99.98 percent). It has an odd number of protons, one, and no neutrons and thus has a magnetic moment, and it is a relatively large one. The oxygen in water is 99 percent ^{16}O, an isotope with an even number of protons and thus no net magnetic moment. The remaining 1 percent of oxygen is either ^{18}O (nonmagnetic) or ^{17}O (magnetic), but it is present at too low a concentration for imaging.

The magnetic moment of the protons in the hydrogen atoms of a water molecule is too small to measure directly in a way that would be useful for imaging. Although their magnetic moments try to orient with the Earth's magnetic field, their thermal motion averages out the magnetic moment of the water molecules in the tissue to zero. A strong external magnetic field will align the magnetic moments, some with the magnetic field and others against it. Slightly more align with the field (lower energy) than against it (higher energy), producing a net magnetic moment in the direction of the applied field. The larger the external field the larger the difference in aligned spins. The Earth's magnetic field strength is between 0.5 and 1.0 gauss (G). In a typical imaging external field of 1 Tesla (1 Tesla [T] = 10,000 G) the excess number of spins in the lower energy state is only three spins per million. In an MRI observation volume equivalent to a pixel in a digital picture (a voxel), three spins per million equals 10^{21} spins, which are enough to detect.

The magnetic moment of the nucleus also experiences a force from the external magnetic field, causing it to precess, rotate like the wobbling of a spinning top, around the direction of the external magnetic field, giving the nucleus a (small) component of magnetization perpendicular to the external magnetic field. The precession is at a frequency dependent on the applied magnetic field and is characteristic of that element's nucleus. There is no overall or net magnetic moment (magnetization) perpendicular to the applied magnetic field because of averaging of the individual nuclei magnetic moments. If an electromagnetic pulse of a frequency that matches the precessional frequency of the nuclei in the sample (for [1]H a frequency in the FM radio frequency range of 42.58 MHz/T of external field strength) is applied perpendicular to the external static magnetic field, the absorbed energy will boost some of the spins from the low-energy spin state (parallel to the external magnetic field) to the high-energy state. When those promoted spins drop back to the lower energy state, they give up that energy as a radiofrequency signal of intensity proportional to the overall magnetic moment, which is detected by a wire coil acting as an antenna. The energy of this transition is very much less than X-rays, 0.6 micro eV (0.6 μeV) compared with a minimum of 100 eV for X-rays. Because the transmitted magnetic signal is small compared with the static magnetic field, the measurement is made at 90 degrees (perpendicular) to the static field after the pulse has been turned off.

For reasons of sensitivity, medical MRI is imaging of the water molecules. Protons that move slowly, such as the protons on collagen, an abundant protein that gives the skin and internal organs their strength and elasticity, give rise to a small magnetic resonance signal that is so spread out over a range of resonant frequencies that it is hardly noticeable in the presence of the much larger amount of liquid water surrounding it. A glass of water does not produce an interesting image because the environment of all the water molecules looks the same (except those at the air-water interface or the walls of the glass). If there were no interaction of the proton magnetization with the environment, the result would be bland for imaging and most other applications. Water in the body looks different because the body has many internal surfaces made of different materials, and spaces filled with fluids of different compositions. The water molecules in these different environments move faster or slower, which affects the way that the magnetic moments of their nuclei interact with magnetic moments of other water molecules or structural elements of the tissue. Hemoglobin combined with oxygen (oxyhemoglobin) in red blood cells is not magnetic, while hemoglobin without oxygen or combined with carbon dioxide is strongly magnetic. The deoxyoxyhemoglobin affects the magnetic moments of the water molecules around those red cells in a way that can be used to generate contrast (can be seen) in a magnetic resonance image. Magnetic resonance signals from the water in less-well-oxygenated blood in vessels show up differently than water near well-oxygenated blood.

Signal received by the wire coil can be decreased in two main ways. They are characterized by the rate constants (or their reciprocals—relaxation times) for how fast they reduce the signal. Microvariations in the local magnetic environment, T2 mechanisms, cause the precessions of the nuclei excited by the radiofrequency (rf) pulse to rapidly fall out of synch with one another reducing the measurable net magnetization perpendicular to the static field. These relaxation mechanisms can be exploited in a variety of ways to obtain specific information about structure and function in tissues. Another mechanism, termed "T1," causes changes in the rate of the return of the net magnetization of the sample by dissipating the absorbed rf energy into modes of molecular vibration and movements of the sample molecules. This energy transfer is most efficient when the collisions or molecular motions occur at frequencies similar to the excitation frequency. Thus, the physical characteristics of the sample strongly influence T1s. For freely diffusing aqueous solutions with little structure such as water or cerebrospinal fluid (CSF), T1s range from 1−4 seconds at 1 T, while for more structured soft tissues, T1s range from 0.1−1 second. Fat has a short T1 (0.241 second), as do skeletal muscle (0.732 second), brain (myelinated) (0.683 second), and brain (unmyelinated) (0.813 second), whereas CSF has a long T1 (2.5 seconds). Measuring signal intensities at appropriately chosen time intervals after excitation would clearly identify differences among these tissues. As an example, fat can be selectively imaged by adjusting the rf pulse sequence and detection parameters. It is the sensitivity and responsiveness of the magnetic resonance signal to both physical and molecular structure that make it so useful for the imaging of soft tissue.

Magnetic resonance imagers utilize a wide variety of ways to obtain magnetic resonance signals that are sensitive to different ways in which the T1 and T2 relaxation rate mechanisms are affected by their environment. These methods are analogous to photographers using different kinds of filters on their camera or using film more sensitive to one portion of the light spectrum than another to enhance particular features of their subject. In magnetic resonance, techniques such as spin echo weighting, T1 weighting, T2 weighting, diffusion tensor imaging, spin density weighting, and other methods designated by exotic acronyms produce images to highlight specific structures, functions, or defects in the tissue or an organ. The signals are obtained by varying the length and spacing of rf pulses, while changing the magnetic field gradients in specific sequences so that resonance signals are detected from protons only in specific types of environment undergoing a particular amount and direction of motion. The sometimes musical and sometimes cacophonous flurry of bangs, clicks, and buzzes that a patient undergoing an MRI procedure hears are a carefully orchestrated series of magnetic field gradient changes and rf pulses to selectively excite and detect protons to generate a particular kind of image. In studies such as blood flow (blood oxygenation level-dependence [BOLD]), the measurement was based on the expected physics from the known biology, but for most other methods, it was a matter of investigators trying different conditions until they got images that best highlighted what they were looking for or suppressed distracting signals. For example, adjusting the data acquisition parameters can make the signals from fat disappear. If only it were that easy for the patient to lose unwanted fat.

ULTRASOUND

Unlike the other modes of medical imaging, ultrasound is not a form of electromagnetic radiation. Sound is a train of pressure or mechanical waves propagating through a compressible medium like a wave on the ocean. Ultrasound is defined as sound with frequencies above 20 kHz (twenty thousand cycles per second). The ability of a physical or electromagnetic wave to interact with an object depends on the size of the object compared with the wavelength of the radiation, that is, the distance between crests (or troughs). Only objects similar in size or larger than that wavelength interact significantly with the wave. Bats can detect small insects with their 100 kHz sonar. At this frequency in air, the sound wavelength is 3.3 mm, which would readily pick up a moth or perhaps a mosquito. In soft tissues of the body, which is predominantly water, sound travels much more rapidly (1,540 meters/second compared with 330 meters/second in air), resulting in a wavelength of 1.54 cm at the bat's frequency of 100 kHz, which would not be useful for many early diagnostic purposes for which millimeter size lesions are expected. For this reason, ultrasound frequencies on the order of megahertz (millions of cycles per second) are used for diagnostic soft tissue imaging. At 2–20 MHz, the most useful frequencies for diagnostic imaging, the wavelengths in water are between 0.77 mm and 0.08 mm, which theoretically can distinguish structures of similar sizes.

High-frequency sound can be generated a variety of ways. A device such as an ultrasonic dog whistle disturbs a high-speed flow of air causing oscillations that are amplified by a resonant chamber. A siren chops airflow into small pieces, which similarly creates high-frequency oscillations. However, the wavelength of the sound produced by these methods is too long to detect what clinicians need to see. A bigger problem is that while a whistle or a siren can be designed to create ultrasound, it is a one-way street. Neither device can receive an ultrasound signal that can be used to create an image. A method was needed to efficiently produce and detect high-frequency (megahertz) oscillations, preferably in the same device.

A seemingly unrelated physics experiment published in 1877 by Jacques Curie and his younger brother Pierre, who was not yet eighteen years old, described the **piezoelectric** (pressure electric) phenomenon exhibited by quartz and certain other materials. Years later Pierre married Marie Sklodowska, forming the husband-wife team that would discover the first naturally radioactive materials, radium and polonium, in 1898. The piezoelectric phenomenon had exactly the property needed for both the production and detection of ultrasound, although that application was many years in the future. An oscillating electrical field induced expansion and contraction cycles in the piezoelectric material and vice versa. The two-way transduction of physical oscillation and electrical oscillations via this phenomenon was rapidly incorporated after its description into microphones, phonographic needle cartridges, and earphones to convert sound waves into electrical currents.

Ultrasound for imaging is generated through a physical effect of an oscillating electrical field operating on a special material, a piezoelectric crystal, periodically changing its physical dimensions. These transducers of electrical energy into mechanical energy include quartz, topaz, calamine, tourmaline, and certain ceramics. Ultrasound transducers currently use synthetic crystals with enhanced properties specially designed for ultrasound work. Oriented dipolar molecules, molecules with a positive charged and a negatively charged end, are formed in a crystal between two plates. When charge is applied to the plates, positive on one plate and negative on the other, the dipolar molecules in the crystal twist slightly to orient in the electrical field. The motion causes the crystal to expand by a few micrometers. Reversing the charge on the plates causes the molecules to twist in the opposite direction contracting the crystal. Cyclic positive and negative charging of the plates at MHz frequencies thus creates a mechanical pressure wave from the crystal expansions and contractions that propagates into the tissue as ultrasound. For pulse operation, the piezoelectric crystal does not have to be excited repeatedly. Like a tuning fork, it has a natural frequency at which it "rings," in which the ultrasound waves reflect back and forth between the front and back of the crystal depending on the distance between the faces. This requires the crystal thickness to be one-half of the chosen ultrasound wavelength. At 1.5 MHz in a typical piezoelectric ceramic such as PZT-5, that wavelength is 2.9 mm, requiring a crystal thickness of 1.45 mm. Because of the difference in the velocity of sound in tissue, this results in an ultrasound beam that has a wavelength and hence a resolving capacity (smallest object observed) of 1 mm.

Sound waves behave physically much like light waves in that they can be focused, reflected, bent (refracted), diffracted, and undergo interference. These properties make them useful for obtaining diagnostic images. Ultrasound has the advantage over visible light in that it readily penetrates the skin (although not bone) and deep into soft tissues. An advantage over X-ray radiation for imaging, besides not being an ionizing form of radiation and thus safer, is that unlike X-rays, ultrasound wavelengths interact with soft tissue in interpretable ways, providing information about its structure and physical state. Many of the methodologies used for forming and manipulating multidimensional images are applicable to ultrasound once the sound waves have been converted into electronic pulses by the receiver. A sound wave, like an ocean wave, displaces molecules of the medium slightly as it passes by a fixed position. Thus, sound waves are sensitive to the physical nature of the medium, including its density and its elasticity or stiffness. Changes in these parameters experienced by the sound wave as it propagates through tissue generate the image. The ultrasound image we see after processing is an image of density or elasticity differences of the surface and internal structures of the tissue that reflect, scatter, or otherwise change the returning signal. By contrast, transmission mode images such as X-ray expend considerable effort (Bucky grid) to remove the relatively small fraction of scattered radiation, which muddies the image by increasing the general background.

Unlike the other forms of imaging considered in this book, ultrasound images are generated from reflected signals rather than from transmitted radiation. This is because ultrasound is lower energy and is readily absorbed by tissue. Absorption of ultrasound increases with increasing frequency and with the shorter wavelengths needed to resolve smaller structures. It is reflected strongly from interfaces between regions of different density or compressibility that transmit too little energy to provide good signal-to-noise for an image in the majority of clinical applications. Interfaces with large differences in the ability to transmit ultrasound are air-liquid and soft tissue-bone. These boundaries obscure any structures beneath them and create artifacts analogous to glare in visible light.

Medical Imaging Timeline

1800	Alessandro Volta constructs first battery.
1820	Hans Christian Oersted describes magnetic effect produced by an electrical current.
1821	Michael Faraday shows that motion can be generated by passing a current in a magnetic field.
1831	Faraday describes magnetic induction.
1831	Joseph Henry invents the electric motor where application of a current in a magnetic field produces motion.
1845	William Thomson develops theory of electromagnetic force.
1865	James Clerk Maxwell develops theory unifying physical phenomena—magnetism and electricity.
1875	William Crookes invents vacuum tube.
1876	Alexander Graham Bell demonstrates first telephone.
1876	Eugen Goldstein discovers cathode rays.
1877	Pierre and Jacques Curie discover piezoelectric effect.
1877	Thomas Edison tests first phonograph.
1880	Crookes shows that cathode rays are electrons, not light.
1883	Edison shows a flow of current from a hot carbon filament to a cold metal wire in an evacuated bulb—the basis for modern electronics.
1887	Heinrich Rudolph Hertz discovers the photoelectric effect.
1888	Hertz produces radio waves.
1888	Frank J. Sprague opens the first electric trolley line, in Richmond, Virginia.

1891	Thomas Edison introduces motion pictures.
1891	George Johnstone Stoney names as yet undiscovered electron.
1891	Almon Stowger patents the automatic telephone exchange.
1892	French physicist Jaques-Arsene d'Arsonval studies the interaction of electromagnetic energy with biological samples; he applies an electromagnetic field to himself and feels warmth but no muscular contraction.
1895	Jean-Baptiste Perrin shows that cathode rays are streams of electrons.
1895	Wilhelm Roentgen discovers X-rays.
1896	Henri Bequerel discovers radioactivity.
1896	General Electric and Siemens begin selling X-ray equipment.
1897	Ernest Rutherford distinguishes between two types of uranium radiation, alpha and beta.
1898	Marie and Pierre Curie discover polonium and radium.
1899	Thomson calculates charge on electron and recognizes that ionization represents splitting of electron from the rest of the atom.
1900	Max Planck proposes that atoms absorb and radiate energy to explain blackbody radiation—the concept of energy quantization.
1900	Paul Ulrich Villard detects gamma rays in radium decay.
1901	Pierre Curie measures heat of radium decay, 110 calories/gram/hour—first example of atomic energy since there was no change in chemical properties.
1901	Hubert Cecil Booth patents the vacuum cleaner.
1902	Rutherford develops transmutation theory of radioactivity.
1903	Wright Brothers take first powered flight at Kitty Hawk, North Carolina.
1904	Thomson proposes model for atom where electrons are embedded in a positive charged atom like raisins in a pound cake.
1904	Charles Glover Barkla determines that the number of charged particles in an atom depends on mass; X-rays are transverse waves like light and thus are electromagnetic.
1906	Barkla reports that more massive elements produce more penetrating X-rays.
1906	Rutherford discovers alpha particle scattering.
1906	Rutherford and Hans Wilhelm Geiger report that alpha particles are related to helium atoms.
1907	Maytag introduces washer.

1908	Ford introduces Model T, costing $850.50.
1908	Geiger counter for the detection of ionizing radiation introduced.
1909	Geiger and Ernest Marsden describe alpha particle scattering by gold foil.
1911	Rutherford proposes model of atom with massive nucleus surrounded by mostly empty space and electrons.
1912	Victor Franz Hess demonstrates the existence of cosmic rays.
1913	Frederick Soddy and Kasimir Fajans propose the radioactive displacement law to account for the loss of mass and electronic charge by radioactive atoms.
1913	Frederick Soddy coins the term "isotope" for atoms of the same element with differing radioactive properties.
1913	Niels Bohr applies quantum theory to the structure of the atom, describing the relationship of electronic orbits and excitation and de-excitation of electrons transitioning between orbits; proposes a solar system-like structural model for the atom.
1913	Henry Mosely demonstrates X-ray spectra of elements.
1913	Gustav Bucky introduces the Bucky Grid to block scattered X-rays, improving image quality.
1913	Albert Salomon documents microcrystals of calcium in breast tumors.
1914	Rutherford names proton.
1917	Paul (Pierre) Langevin develops sonar.
1921	Air contrast myelinography improves images of the nerve channel in the spinal column.
1923	Louis deBroglie proposes theory of wave-particle duality of matter.
1925	Werner Heisenberg introduces matrix mechanics.
1926	Erwin Schroedinger proposes wave mechanics.
1926	Enrico Fermi describes quantum statistics.
1927	Heisenberg proposes uncertainty principle.
1930	Paul Dirac develops equation for relativistic electrons, predicts the existence of the positive electron—the positron.
1930	Allesandro Vallebona mechanically links motion of X-ray tube and film around the patient to isolate specific image information producing the first tomographic images.
1931	John Cockcroft and Ernest Walton study nuclear reactions with proton beams.

1932	Carl D. Anderson reports observation of the positron.
1932	James Chadwick adds the neutron as a component of the nucleus.
1933	Fermi proposes theory of beta decay.
1934	Marie Curie dies from leukemia caused by her radiation exposure.
1935	George Hevesy shows that certain natural radioisotopes are retained or concentrated in specific tissues or organs.
1938	Lise Meitner and Otto Fritsch propose theory of fission.
1939	Niels Bohr and John Wheeler propose theory of fission.
1946	Edward Purcell and Felix Bloch report the measurement of the radiofrequency response of water protons in a magnetic field.
1953	Real-time ultrasound imaging captures the heart in motion.
1954	Ultrasound is applied in gynecology and obstetrics.
1958	William Oldendorf constructs a computed tomography (CT) scanner without computer.
1963	Alan Cormack applies a line-integral method to reconstruct a two-dimensional image from a CT scan utilizing a computer.
1967	Charles M. Gros develops the first dedicated radiological equipment for mammography.
1970	Hank Anger develops SPECT scanner.
1971	Goeffrey Hounsfield applies first commercial CT scanner (EMI) and first clinical use to detect a brain tumor.
1971	First image is obtained by magnetic resonance (called NMR).
1972	Raymond Damadian files for patent on NMR as a diagnostic method for cancer.
1972	Michael M. Ter-Pogossian's "lead chicken" produces crude PET image.
1973	Paul Lauterbur publishes first image using NMR, a technique he names zeugmatography.
1975	Michel M. Ter-Pogossian, Michael E. Phelps, and E. J. Hofman describe a scanner for PET imaging.
1975	Ultrasound becomes commercially successful.
1977	Raymond Damadian builds a whole-body MRI scanner he names *Indomitable*.
1977	Peter Mansfield develops echoplanar method of collecting MRI data to allow fast acquisition to measure motion and acquire three-dimensional images.
1979	Fluorine-18 (labeled FDG) is synthesized and used for PET imaging of brain glucose metabolism.

1985   Food and Drug Administration removes its label of "experimental procedure" from MRI, allowing reimbursement by Medicare and private insurers.

1991   Seiji Ogawa demonstrates areas of increased metabolic activity in the brain with his blood oxygenation level-dependent (BOLD) MRI method.

1996   M. C. Preul uses MRS imaging to diagnose brain tumors.

Glossary

algorithm A mathematical calculation performed on imaging data to generate an image.

ampere A unit of the amount of an electrical current.

Anger camera Multidetector scintillation camera designed by Hal Anger to detect gamma photons and create an image.

angiography Visualization of integrity of blood vessels by the introduction of X-ray absorbing contrast agent.

annihilation Interaction of normal matter and antimatter (electron and positron) converting their mass into two 0.511 MeV gamma photons.

anode Positive electrode—accepts electrons.

antimatter Form of matter with opposite characteristics from normal matter. When antimatter comes in contact with its normal counterpart they annihilate each other, creating a large amount of energy.

arteriogram Visualization of blood vessels.

atomic number Number of protons in the nucleus of an atom of an element.

back projection Mathematical processing to recreate an image from the radiation emanating from the subject.

bioelectricity Electrical currents produced by living cells and tissues as a result of the flow of ions.

bioimpedance The interaction of externally applied electrical currents and their accompanying magnetic fields with an organism. This is distinguished from bioelectricity, which is endogenously generated electrical currents.

bremsstrahlung X-ray radiation released when a high-speed free electron is deflected (scattered) by the orbital electrons of an atom.

cathode Negative electrode—supplies electrons.

cathode rays Term used to describe energy emitted from a cathode before they were characterized and named electrons.

cerebrospinal fluid Transparent body fluid bathing the brain and the spinal cord.

collimator Lead dividers separating detector elements to restrict the field of view of the elements to incoming photons traveling parallel to the collimator walls.

color encoding Method of indicating signal intensity using color: red for high, green for medium, and blue or black for low.

Compton camera A radiation detector that combines Compton scattering and scintillation detection to trace the position of the origin of a single gamma photon in a patient.

contrast agent Material introduced into subject when imaging to more clearly distinguish features from surrounding tissue.

Coolidge tube A more efficient tube for X-ray production that used direct electrical current rather than alternating current; designed by William Coolidge.

coronal section Series of sections running from top to bottom.

Cost-benefit analysis Cost utility plus pain plus inconvenience. This type of analysis is not considered appropriate for ethical reasons because it puts a monetary value on life.

Cost-effective analysis Gain in health compared to the cost of obtaining that gain. Cost per year of life gained. Cost per quality-adjusted year of life gained.

Cost-utility analysis Adjustments made for "value attached to the benefits."

Crookes tube First X-ray source made of thin glass and containing two electrodes sealed into a vacuum. When the electrodes were charged the tube emitted X-rays.

crystallography Structure determination of molecules in a crystal by diffraction of (usually) X-rays. The structure is back-calculated from the pattern of scattered X-rays.

cyclotron A device in which electrons, protons, and other charged species could be accelerated to high energies and collided with a target to produce nuclear reactions. Positron-emitting radioactive isotopes are produced in this way without requiring a nuclear reactor.

DICOM Digital Imaging and Communications in Medicine; an electronic communications protocol for exchanging digital information including medical images.

diffraction Deflection of radiation by its interaction with matter.

Doppler echocardiography Determination of the speed and direction of blood flow by the changes in the ultrasound frequency (Doppler shift) scattered from moving red blood cells.

electrocardiogram Recording of the electrical activity of heart muscle in the cardiac cycle as it beats.

electroencephalogram (EEG) Recording of nerve activity in the brain.

electromagnetic radiation Sinusoidally varying electrical fields and their corresponding magnetic fields moving through space. The concept of wave-particle duality emphasizes that this energy can alternatively be thought of as particle-like or wave-like in different situations.

electromyography Recording of the electrical activity of skeletal muscle.

electron Negatively charged particle that orbits the nucleus of an atom.

electron paramagnetic resonance (EPR) Absorbance of a radiofrequency by the magnetic moment of an unpaired electron of an atom or molecule in a magnetic field.

electroneurography Recording of the electrical activity of a nerve, often a nerve connected to a muscle.

embolism Blood vessel blockage.

endorphin Normal (endogenous) pain-blocking peptides produced by the body that act like opiate pain-killing drugs.

endoscopy Visible light imaging of internal body cavities through an inserted physical probe.

erythema dose A crude estimation of the biological effect of a dose of ionizing radiation defined as the amount of radiation sufficient to cause reddening of (Caucasian) skin.

FDG PET-labeled glucose analog used to measure metabolic activity.

fluorescence Reradiation of energy from an electronic state excited by absorption of a photon. Emission occurs at a longer wavelength (lower energy) than the incident photon.

fluoroscope Real-time method of viewing X-ray absorption of a subject using a screen that emits light when struck by X-ray photons rather than film. Phosphor screens have been replaced by image-intensifying devices that multiply the light intensity many thousand-fold.

Geiger-Muller tube Gas-filled tube that detects ionization events caused by high-energy radiation.

grazing-angle reflection Method of focusing X-rays, which penetrate most materials, by directing the beam at a shallow angle barely skimming the surface to change the direction of the X-rays by a small amount.

half-life Time required for one-half of the atoms of a radioactive atom to decay.

heat plot Display of signal intensity by color-encoding.

ion channel Protein in a cell membrane containing a channel through which ions flow through the ion-impermeable lipid bilayer.

isotope Form of an element in which the nucleus has a different number of neutrons than protons.

kernel Mathematical term that describes a computation.

ligand Molecule that binds to (usually) a protein that elicits a response. Hormone receptors and ion channels bind ligands that change those protein's activities. Monitoring of the amount and the location of the binding of radio-labeled versions of ligands can be monitored by PET or SPECT to determine the amount and location of the ligand's receptor.

mammography X-ray imaging of the breast.

metabonomics Study of the molecules present in a cell or tissue in a particular metabolic state. Magnetic resonance spectroscopy can be used to detect the different molecules and to determine changes in their relative amounts in a diseased state or after treatment.

multiplanar reconstruction Computerized stacking of two-dimensional sections to create a three-dimensional image.

myelinography Visualization of the integrity of nerve tracts and myelin sheaths by medical imaging technology.

neurotransmitter Chemical released by a neuron as a result of an action potential that crosses the gap (synaptic cleft) between neurons to bind to a receptor protein and trigger a response in the next neuron in the pathway.

nuclear imaging Imaging using gamma-emitting radioisotopes.

PACS Picture Archiving and Communications Systems; suite of medical systems hardware and software that actually run digital medical imaging including data acquisition, archiving images, and display and manipulation systems.

paramagnetism Magnetism caused by one or more unpaired electron spins in an atom or molecule.

piezoelectric Property of certain materials such as quartz to produce an electrical current when compressed or expanded (pressure-electric).

pixel Smallest digital element in a two-dimensional image.

positron Antiparticle of the electron, sometimes referred to as a "positively charged electron."

QALY Quality-adjusted life year; increase in life expectancy provided by a diagnostic therapeutic intervention adjusted for improvement in function and decrease in discomfort or pain.

radioisotope An isotope whose neutron composition makes it energetically unstable and liable to rearrange emitting electromagnetic radiation and/or subatomic particles.

radionuclide Radioactive isotope of an element.

radiopharmaceutical Drug with a radioactive tracer atom incorporated into its structure.

reconstruction Computational method of formation of an image from the back-projected paths of the photons of the type of radiation employed in the imaging.

Roentgen rays Name given in Germany to the emissions Roentgen called X-rays.

sagittal Lengthwise side to side.

single photon emission imaging Imaging modality that uses radioisotopes that decay via emission of a single gamma-ray photon.

spiral CT Rapid X-ray computed tomography imaging technique in which the subject is moved in a straight line through the center of a rotating X-ray source and camera such that the two-dimensional "slices" stack to form a helix or spiral rather than a loaf of bread.

SQUID Super-conducting quantum interference device.

Superconductivity Condition of an electrical conductor in which all electrical resistance disappears. An electric current flowing in a semiconducting loop would theoretically continue to circulate forever. Present superconduictors require ultra-low temperatures (near absolute zero, 0°K).

Tesla Unit of magnetic field strength = 10,000 gauss = 20,000 × the Earth's magnetic field.

test phantom An object made of patterns of materials that interact with a particular form of imaging radiation to different extents. It is used to evaluate performance of the instrumentation such as resolution and density differences similar to the objects being imaged and provide a measure of quality control of both the equipment and the computational algorithms.

tomography From the Greek *tomos* meaning section, slice, or cut. Images are two-dimensional, representing absorption or emission from within a defined thickness of the subject. Sections are stacked to reconstruct a three-dimensional picture.

ultrasonography Imaging with ultrasound energy. The image is formed from reflected ultrasound waves with the depth within the subject represented by the time delay between emission of an ultrasound pulse and its reception.

volt A unit for measurement of the force of an electrical current.

voxel An observation volume; a unit used in MRI, PET, and SPECT imaging to define the smallest unit of an image, analogous to a pixel of a two-dimensional digital image.

wavelength Distance between wave crests for electromagnetic radiation and ultrasound.

zeugmatography From the Greek *zeugma*—"to join together." Term given by Paul Lauterbur to describe the interaction of the magnetic field gradient and radiofrequency resonance he used to locate the position of a resonance in a subject to produce magnetic resonance images.

REFERENCES AND FURTHER READING

REFERENCES

Beinfield, M. T. "Cost-effectiveness of Whole-body CT Screening." *Radiology* 234 (2005):415–422.

Brecher, R., and E. Brecher. *The Rays: A History of Radiology in the United States and Canada.* Baltimore, MD: Williams and Wilkins, 1969.

Brenner, D. J., and C. D. Elliston. "Estimated Radiation Risks Potentially Associated with Full-body CT Screening." *Radiology* 232 (2004):735–738.

Chapman D., W. Thomlinson, R. E. Johnston, D. Washburn, E. Pisano, N. Gmur, Z. Zhong, R. Menk, F. Arfelli, and D. Sayers. "Diffraction Enhanced X-Ray Imaging." *Physics in Medicine and Biology* 42 (1997):2015–2025.

Cho, M. K. "Understanding Incidental Findings in the Context of Genetics and Genomics." *Journal of Law, Medicine and Ethics* 36 (2008):280–285.

Chrysanthou, M. "Transparency and Selfhood: Utopia and the Informed Body." *Social Science and Medicine* 54 (2002):469–479.

Dilmanian, F. A., Z. Zhong, B. Ren, X. Y. Wu, L. D. Chapman, I. Orion, and W. C. Thomlinson. "Computed Tomography of X-Ray Index of Refraction Using the Diffraction Enhanced Imaging Method." *Physics in Biology and Medicine* 45 (2000):933–946.

Doby, T., and G. Alker. *Origins and Development of Medical Imaging.* Carbondale: Southern Illinois University Press, 1997.

Ehrlich, P. *Deutsche Medizinische Wochenschrift* 12 (1886):19–52.

Engelmann, J., J. Bacelo, M. Metzen, R. Pusch, B. Bouton, A. Migliaro, A. Caputi, R. Budelli, K. Grant, and G. von der Emde. "Electric Imaging through Active Electrolocation: Implication for the Analysis of Complex Scenes." *Biological Cybernetics* 98 (2008):519–539.

Etcoff, N. L., P. Ekman, J. J. Magee, and M. G. Frank. "Lie Detection and Language Comprehension." *Nature* 405 (2000):139.

FDA (Food and Drug Administration). "Radiation Emitting Products/Radiation Emitting Products and Procedures." Available at http://www.fda.gov/RadiationEmittingProducts/RadiationEmittingProductsandProcedures (accessed August 10, 2009).

Finkel, M. L. *Understanding the Mammography Controversy: Science, Politics, and Breast Cancer Screening.* Westport, CT: Praeger, 2005.

Furtado, C. D., D. A. Aguirre, and C. B. Se. "Whole-body CT Screening: Spectrum of Findings and Recommendations in 1192 Patients." *Radiology* 237 (2005):385−394.

Glasser, O. *Dr. W. C. Roentgen.* Springfield, IL: Charles C. Thomas, 1945.

Golan, T. "The Emergence of the Silent Witness: The Legal and Medical Reception of X-Rays in the USA." *Social Studies of Science* 34 (2004):469−499.

Granot, Y., A. Ivorra, and B. Rubinsky. "A New Concept for Medical Imaging Centered on Cellular Phone Technology." *PLoS ONE* 3, no. 4 (2008): e2075

Henschke, C. I., D. I. McCauley, D. F. Yankelevitz, D. P. Naidich, G. McGuiness, O. S. Miettinen, D. Libby, M. W. Pasmantier, J. Koizumi, N. K. Altorki, and J. P. Smith. "Early Lung Cancer Action Project: Overall Design and Findings from Baseline Screening." *Lancet* 354 (1999): 99−105.

Hoaglin, M., A. Eifler, A. McDermott, E. Motan, and P. Beithon. "Integrated Digital X-Ray System for the WHIS-RAD." *Africa Field Report*: Northwestern University/University of Cape Town, Biomedical Engineering Department for Rotary International, 2006.

Illes, J., M. P. Kirschen, E. Edwards, L. R. Stanford, P. Bandettini, M. K. Cho, P. J. Ford, G. H. Glover, J. Kulynych, R. Macklin, D. B. Michael, and S. M. Wolf. "Incidental Findings in Brain Imaging Research." *Science* 311 (2006):783−784.

Inglehart, J. K. "The New Era of Medical Imaging: Progress and Pitfalls." *New England Journal of Medicine* 354, no. 26 (2006):2822−2828.

Kevles, B. "Body Imaging: How Doctors Learned to Peer Beneath Our Skin to See What Might Be Wrong without Using Surgery." *Newsweek* 130, no. 24-A (1997):74−76.

Kevles, B. *Naked to the Bone: Medical Imaging in the 20th Century.* Cambridge, MA: Perseus Publishers, 1998.

Kleinfield, S. *A Machine Called Indomitable.* New York: Time Books, 1985.

Kozel, F. A., K. A. Johnson, Q. Mu, E. L. Grenesko, S. J. Laken, and M. S. George. "Detecting Deception Using Functional Magnetic Resonance Imaging." *Biological Psychiatry* 58, no. 8 (2005):605−613.

Kulich, R., R. Maciewicz, and S. J. Scrivani. "Functional Magnetic Resonance Imaging (fMRI) and Expert Testimony." *Pain Medicine* 10, no. 2 (2009):373−380.

Langelben, D. D. "Detection of Deception with fMRI: Are We There Yet?" *Legal and Criminological Psychology* 13, no. 1 (2008):1−9.

Langelben, D. D., J. W. Loughead, W. B. Bilker, K. Ruparel, A. R. Childress, S. I. Busch, and R. C. Gur. "Telling Truth from Lie in Individual Subjects with Fast Event-related fMRI." *Human Brain Mapping* 26, no. 4 (2005):262–272.

Lee, T. H., and T. A. Brennan. "Direct-to-Consumer Marketing of High-Technology Screening Tools." *New England Journal of Medicine* 346, no. 7 (2002):529–531.

Marano, L. "Ethics and Mapping the Brain." *Washington Times*, June 3, 2003.

Mayo, T. W., and T. E. Kepler. *Telemedicine: Survey and Analysis of Federal and State Laws*. Washington, DC: American Health Lawyers Association, 2007.

Medical Imaging Technology Roadmap Steering Committee. "Future Needs for Medical Imaging in Health Care. Report of Working Group 1." In *Medical Imaging Technology Roadmap*. Industry Ottawa: Ontario Canada: Industry Canada, 2000.

Moriarty, J. C. "Flickering Admissibility: Neuroimaging Evidence in the U.S. Courts." *Behavioral Sciences and the Law* 26 (2008):29–49.

Moser, J. W. "The Deficit Reduction Act of 2005: Policy, Politics, and Impact on Radiologists." *Journal of the American College of Radiology* 3 (2006):744–750.

National Center for Health Statistics. *Health United States, 2008*. Hyattsville, MD: Centers for Disease Control and Prevention, 2008.

New South Wales Government Department of Environment CCaW. "Information on Whole Body Scanning," 2008. Available at http://www.environ ment.nsw.gov.au/radiation/ctbodyscans.htm (accessed August 10, 2009).

Oldendorf, W. H. *The Quest for an Image of the Brain*. New York: Raven Press, 1980.

Parham, C., Z. Zhong, D. M. Connor, L. D. Chapman, and E. D. Pisano. "Design and Implementation of a Compact Low-Dose Diffraction Enhanced Medical Imaging System." *Academic Radiology* 16 (2009):911–917.

Perry, J. E., L. R. Churchill, and H. S. Kirshner. "The Terri Schiavo Case: Legal, Ethical, and Medical Perspectives." *Annals of Internal Medicine* 143 (2005):744–748.

Pusch, R., G. Von der Emde, M. Hollmann, J. Bacelo, S. Nobel, K. Grant, and J. Engelmann. "Active Sensing in a Mormyrid Fish: Electric Images and Peripheral Modifications of the Signal Carrier Give Evidence of Dual Foveation." *Journal of Experimental Biology* 211 (2008):921–934.

Regge, D., C. Laudi, G. Galatola, P. D. Monica, L. Bonelli, G. Angelelli, R. Asnaghi, B. Barbaro, C. Bartolozzi, D. Bielen, L. Boni, C. Borghi, P. Bruzzi, M. C. Cassinis, M. Galia, T. M. Gallo, A. Grasso, C. Hassan, A. Laghi, M. C. Martina, E. Neri, C. Senore, G. Simonetti, S. Venturini, and G. Gandini. "Diagnostic Accuracy of Computed Tomographic Colonography for the Detection of Advanced Neoplasia in Individuals at Increased Risk of Colorectal Cancer." *JAMA* 301 (2009):2453–2461.

Rosner, F. *Medicine in the Bible and the Talmud*. New York: Yeshiva University Press, 1977.

Sanger, C. "Seeing and Believing: Mandatory Ultrasound and the Path to a Protected Choice." *UCLA Law Review* 56 (2008):351–408.

Scarborough, J. "Celsus on Human Vivisection in Ptolemaic Alexandria." *Clio Medicine* 11 (2008):2538.

Schinzel, B. "The Body in Medical Imaging between Reality and Construction." *Poiesis Prax* 4 (2006):185−198.

Stoddard, P. K., and M. R. Markham. "Signal Cloaking by Electric Fish." *Bioscience* 58, no. 5 (2008):415−425.

Taylor, J. S. "Image of Contradiction: Obstetrical Ultrasound in American Culture." In *Reproducing Reproduction: Kinship, Power, and Technological Innovation*, Vol. 15, eds. S. Franklin, and H. Ragone. Philadelpha, PA: University of Pennsylvania Press, 1998.

Taylor, J. S. "The Public Life of the Fetal Sonogram and the Work of the Sonographer." *Journal of Diagnostic Medical Sonography* 367 (2002):368−369.

U.S. GAO (U.S. Government Accountability Office). *MEDICARE PART B IMAGING SERVICES. Rapid Spending Growth and Shift to Physician Offices Indicate Need for CMS to Consider Additional Management Practices.* Washington, DC: Government Printing Office, 2008.

U.S. Preventive Services Task Force. "Screening for Breast Cancer: Recommendations and Rationale." *Annals of Internal Medicine* 137 (2002): 34446.

U.S. Preventive Services Task Force. "Screening for Breast Cancer: U.S. Preventive Services Task Force Recommendation Statement." *Annals of Internal Medicine* 151 (2009): 71626.

United States Office for the Advancement of Telehealth. *2001 Telemedicine Report to Congress.* Washington, DC: U.S. Department of Health and Human Services, Health Resources and Services Administration, 2001.

Valk, P. E., D. L. Bailey, D. W. Townsend, and M. N. Maisey. *Positron Emission Tomography: Basic Science and Clinical Practice.* London: Springer-Verlag, 2003.

van Dijck, J. *The Transparent Body: A Cultural Analysis of Medical Imaging,* eds. P. Thurtle, and R. Mitchell. Seattle: University of Washington Press, 2005.

Vrij, A. *Detecting Lies and Deceit: The Psychology of Lying and the Implications for Professional Practice.* Chichester, UK: England Wiley, 2001.

Weinstein, M. C., J. E. Siegel, M. R. Gold, M. S. Kamlet, and L. B. Russell. "Recommendations of the Panel on Cost-effectiveness in Health and Medicine." *JAMA* 276, no. 15 (1996):1253−1258.

Wilkens, L. A., and M. H. Hofmann. "The Paddlefish Rostrum as an Electrosensory Organ: A Novel Adaptation for Plankton Feeding." *Bioscience* 57, no. 5 (2007):399−407.

Withers, S. "The Story of the First Roentgen Evidence." *Radiology* 19 (1931):99−100.

Wolf, S. M., F. P. Lawrenz, C. A. Nelson, J. P. Kahn, M. K. Cho, E. W. Clayton, J. G. Fletcher, M. K. Georgieff, D. Hammerschmidt, K. Hudson, J. Illes, V. Kapur, M. A. Keane, B. A. Koenig, B. S. LeRoy, E. G. McFarland,

J. Paradise, L. S. Parker, S. F. Terry, B. V. Ness, and B. S. Wilfond. "Managing Incidental Findings in Human Subjects Research: Analysis and Recommendations." *Journal of Law and Medical Ethics* 36 (2008):219–248.

WHIA (World Heath Imaging Alliance) and SIIM (Society for Imaging Informatics in Medicine). "World Health Imaging Alliance (WHIA) Announces Support from the Society for Imaging Informatics in Medicine (SIIM)." 2009. Available at http://www.worldhealthimaging.org/documents/WHIA SIIMPressReleasefinal.pdf (accessed January 28, 2010).

WHO (World Health Organization). *Essential Health Technologies Strategy 2004–2007.* Geneva, Switzerland: World Health Organization, 2003.

WHO (World Health Organization). *Essential Diagnostic Imaging, 2009.* Geneva, Switzerland: World Health Organization, 2009.

Yelin, D., I. Rizvi, W. M. White, J. T. Motz, T. Hasan, B. E. Bouma, and G. J. Tearney. "Three-dimensional Miniature Endoscopy." *Nature* 443 (2006): 765.

Yelin, D., W. M. White, J. T. Motz, S. H. Yun, and B. E. Bouma. "Spectral-domain Spectrally-encoded Endoscopy." *Optics Express* 15 (2007):2433–2444.

Zaidi, H. "Medical Physics in Developing Countries: Looking for a Better World." *Biomedical Imaging and Intervention Journal* 4, no. 1 (2008):e29.

FURTHER READING

Adam, A., A. K. Dixon, R. G. Grainger, and D. J. Allison. *Grainger & Allison's Diagnostic Radiology: A Textbook of Medical Imaging*, 5th ed., 2 vols. Philadelphia, PA: Churchill Livingstone/Elsevier, 2008.

Allison, W. *Fundamental Physics for Probing and Imaging.* New York: Oxford University Press, 2006.

Baker, C. W. *Scientific Visualization.* Brookfield, CT: Millbrook Press, 2000.

Bernstein L. *The Transparent Body.* Middletown, CT: Wesleyan University Press, 1989.

Brecher, R., and E. Brecher. *The Rays: A History of Radiology in the United States and Canada.* Baltimore, MD: Williams and Wilkins, 1969.

Brezinski, M. E. *Optical Coherance Tomography: Principles and Applications.* New York: Elsevier Science and Technical Books, 2006.

Brodwin, P. E., ed. *Biotechnology and Culture: Bodies, Anxieties, Ethics.* Bloomington: Indiana University Press, 2000.

Burrows, E. H. *Pioneers and Early Years: A History of British Radiology.* Alderney, UK: Colophon, 1986.

Bushberg, J. T. *The Essential Physics of Medical Imaging*, 2nd ed. Philadelphia: Lippincott Williams & Wilkins, 2002.

Cronan, J. J. "History of Venous Ultrasound." *Journal of Ultrasound in Medicine* 22 (2003):1143–1146.

DeGraaf, R. *In vivo NMR Spectroscopy: Principles and Techniques*, 2nd ed. New York: Wiley and Sons, 2008.

Doby, T., and G. Alker. *Origins and Development of Medical Imaging*. Carbondale: Southern Illinois University Press, 1997.

Doi, K. "Computer-aided Diagnosis in Medical Imaging: Historical Review, Current Status and Future Potential." *Computerized Medical Imaging and Graphics* 31, no. 4–5 (2007):198–211.

Ehrlich, R. A., and J. A. Daly. *Patient Care in Radiography: With an Introduction to Medical Imaging*, 7th ed. St. Louis, MO: Mosby Elsevier, 2009.

Epstein, C. L. *Introduction to the Mathematics of Medical Imaging*. Upper Saddle River, NJ: Pearson Education, 2003.

Finkel, Madelon L. *Understanding the Mammography Controversy: Sceince, Politics, and Breast Cancer Screening*. Westport, CT: Praeger, 2005.

Gherman, B. *The Mysterious Rays of Dr. Roentgen*. New York: Atheneum, 1994.

Goldsmith, B. *Obsessive Genious. The Inner World of Marie Curie*. New York: Norton, 2005.

Grimnes, S., and O. G. Martinsen. *Bioimpedance and Bioelectricity Basics*. New York: Academic Press, 2000.

Hedrick, W. R., D. L. Hykes, and D. E. Starchman. *Ultrasound Physics and Instrumentation*, 4th ed. New York: Elsevier, 2005.

Hendee, W. R., and Ritenour, E. R. *Medical Imaging Physics*, 4th ed. New York: Wiley-Liss, 2002.

Holder, D. S. *Electrical Impedance Tomography: History and Applications*. Melville, NY: American Institute of Physics, 2004.

Isherwood, I. "Sir Godfrey Hounsfield." *Radiology* 234, no. 3 (2005):975.

Kevles, B. *Naked to the Bone: Medical Imaging in the 20th Century*: New York: Perseus Publishers, 1998.

Kleinfield, S. *A Machine Called Indomitable*. New York: Time Books, 1985.

Macchia, R. J., J. E. Termine, C. D. Buchen, V. Raymond, and M. D. Damadian. "Magnetic Resonance Imaging and the Controversy of the 2003 Nobel Prize in Physiology or Medicine." *Journal of Urology* 178 (2007):783–785.

Mattson, J. S., and M. Simon. *The Pioneers of NMR and Magnetic Resonance in Medicine: The Story of MRI*. New York: Bar-Ilan University Press, 1996.

McClafferty, C. K. *The Head Bone's Connected to the Neck Bone: The Weird and Wonderful X-Ray*. New York: Farrar, Straus, and Giraud, 2001.

Meyer-Bäse, A. *Pattern Recognition For Medical Imaging*. Amsterdam and Boston: Elsevier Academic Press, 2004.

Morgagni, J. B. *The Seats and Causes of Disease Investigated by Anatomy*, trans. B. Alexander Birmingham, AL: Classics of Medicine Library, 1983.

Oldendorf, W. H. *The Quest for an Image of the Brain*. New York: Raven Press, 1980.

Ordidge, R. "The Development of Echo-planar Imaging (EPI): 1977–1982." *MAGMA* 9 (1999):117–121.

Patton, D. D. "The Birth of Nuclear Medicine Instrumentation: Blumgart and Yens, 1925." *Journal of Nuclear Medicine* 44 (2003):1362–1365.

Peters, T. M. "From Radio-astronomy to Medical Imaging." *Australasian Physical & Engineering Sciences in Medicine* 14 (1991):185–188.

Porter, R. *The Greatest Benefit to Mankind. A Medical History of Humanity.* New York: W. W. Norton, 1997.

Ring, E. F. "The Historical Development of Thermal Imaging in Medicine." *Rheumatology (Oxford)* 43, no. 6 (2004):800–802.

Rothenberg, L. N., and A. G. Haus. "Physicists in Mammography—A Historical Perspective." *Medical Physics* 22 (1995):1923–1934.

Sherry, C. J., and R. S. Ledley. *Medical Imaging Careers.* New York: VGM Career Books, 2000.

Sickles, E. A. "Breast Imaging: From 1965 to the Present." *Radiology* 215 (2000):1–16.

Sprawls, P. *Physical Principles of Medical Imaging*, 2nd ed. Gaithersburg, MD: Aspen Publishers, 1993.

Swanson, D. P., H. M. Chilton, and J. H. Thrall. *Pharmaceuticals in Medical Imaging: Radiopaque Contrast Media, Radiopharmaceuticals, Enhancement Agents For Magnetic Resonance Imaging and Ultrasound.* New York: Macmillan Pub. Co., 1990.

U.S. Preventive Services Task Force. "Screening for Breast Cancer: Recommendations and Rationale." *Annals of Internal Medicine* 137 (2002): 344–46.

U.S. Preventive Services Task Force. "Screening for Breast Cancer: U.S. Preventive Services Task Force Recommendation Statement." *Annals of Internal Medicine* 151 (2009): 716–26.

Valk, P. E., D. L. Bailey, D. W. Townsend, and M. N. Maisey. *Positron Emission Tomography. Basic Science and Clinical Practice.* London: Springer-Verlag, 2003.

van Dijck, J. *The Transparent Body: A Cultural Analysis of Medical Imaging.* Ed. P. Thurtle, and R. Mitchell. Seattle: University of Washington Press, 2005.

Webb, S. *The Physics of Medical Imaging.* New York: Taylor and Francis, 2008.

Wilson, B. G. *Ethics and Basic Law for Medical Imaging Professionals.* Philadelphia: F.A. Davis Co., 1997.

Wolbarst, A. B. *Looking Within: How X-ray, CT, MRI, Ultrasound, and Other Medical Images Are Created and How They Help Physicians to Save Lives.* Berkeley: University of California Press, 1999.

Zannos, S. *Godfrey Hounsfield and the Invention of CAT Scans.* Bear, DE: Mitchell Lane Publishers, 2003.

INDEX